DONOR CONCEPTION

A step-by-step guide

DONOR CONCEPTION

A step-by-step guide

FEATURES AUSTRALIAN POLICIES AND LEGISLATION

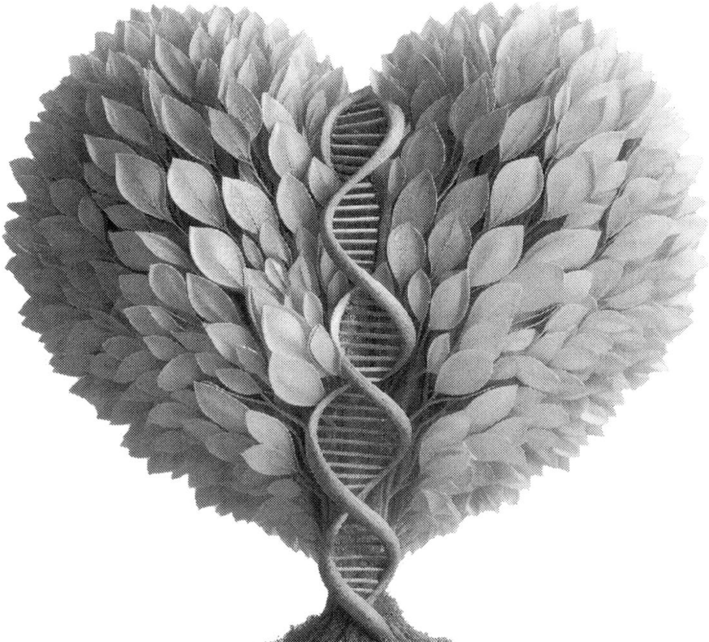

Gail Pascoe

GLP
PUBLISHING

Published by GLP Publishing
info@donorconceptionandbeyond.com.au

First published 2024

Cover image created with the assistance of DALL·E 2
Typeset in Heuristica 10pt and Fira Sans
Printed in Australia

ISBN: 978-0-646-89426-3 (Paperback)
ISBN: 978-0-646-89427-0 (e-Book)

NATIONAL LIBRARY OF AUSTRALIA

A catalogue record for this book is available from the National Library of Australia

Disclaimers
The URLs in this book were current at the time of publication. The author and publisher are unable to guarantee the ongoing currency of any URLs appearing in this book.

Obituary
Gail Pascoe, loving and much loved mother, daughter, sister, and friend, passed away on 17 May 2024, just days before the publication of this book—her life's legacy to her beautiful daughter. Inspired by her own journey to motherhood, Gail's hopes for this book were that it would be a resource for every person wishing to become a parent through donor conception.

To my beautiful angel.
Without you this book would not exist.
I love you forever.

Foreword

In this profoundly insightful and thoroughly detailed book, Gail Pascoe captures the intricate journey of donor conception with the sensitivity it demands. Drawing from her personal experience as a single mother and the nuanced perspectives of her donor-conceived daughter, she offers a guiding light to prospective recipient parents.

This book delves into the ethical considerations and emotional complexities of donor conception, urging parents to place the well-being and identity of donor-conceived children at the forefront of their decisions.

A must-read for anyone involved in or considering donor conception, it provides invaluable lessons on respecting and honouring the unique stories of these children, ultimately shaping a more thoughtful and informed approach to modern family building.

Jana Rupnow*, MA, LPC
Janarupnow.com

* Jana Rupnow is the author of *Three makes baby: How to parent your donor-conceived child.*[1]

Contents

Disclaimer

The author has made every attempt to ensure the accuracy and reliability of the information in this book and all information is considered to be true and correct at the time of publication; changes in circumstance over which the author has no control after publication may impact upon the accuracy of the material. The author assumes no responsibility for errors, inaccuracies, omissions or any other inconsistencies herein.

This book is intended solely as a source of information and general guidance and is not intended to constitute health advice nor to act in any way as a substitute for consultation with a competent, qualified, professional and licensed health practitioner. Please consult with your own healthcare specialist before making important personal decisions.

It is not intended as a definitive set of instructions. Furthermore, any of the author's personal views and opinions expressed herein are solely the author's own views and opinions and are also not intended to be treated as a definitive set of instructions. The author, publisher and all contracted publishing professionals cannot be held liable for issues associated with readers acting upon any information in this book. No legal liability will be accepted for any loss, injury or damage that may occur due to reliance on anything stated herein.

This book is not intended to constitute legal advice or any other advice of a professional nature. If you require legal or other professional advice and/or assistance, please consult with your own legal or professional advisor to discuss the facts and circumstances that apply to you prior to making important personal decisions.

Acknowledgments

I've always wanted to be a writer and completed my first novella when I was eleven—a work of fiction called *A Bloody Murder*. A lot more swearing was involved in the ten years it took to complete this book and, I confess, I truly had no idea how difficult it would be to get a book done, dusted and published. I am now in complete awe of every writer who has ever done so.

Ten years is a long time, so there are many people to thank.

I want to start by expressing my eternal gratitude to all the people who supplied quotes for this book. Your direct experiences and words of wisdom have added a richness I could never have provided alone. To all the intended and recipient parents, the donors, and *especially* the donor-conceived individuals who generously shared their words, thank you from the bottom of my heart. I want to particularly acknowledge those for whom providing help for me brought up all kinds of raw emotions and grief, yet they chose to support me anyway. Thank you!

I am indebted to all my amazing beta readers who read this thing from end to end and gave me the most incredible feedback and suggestions for making this book the best it could be. Thank you to Kate Bourne, Jana Rupnow, Ian Smith, Alana McDonald, Hayley Smith, Beth Wright, Aimee Shackleton, Ashley Ford, Ell Meghan Bell, Valerie Lyrics and the rest of you who don't wish to be named.

A very special thanks must also go to Donor Conceived Australia for your unending support and guidance regarding all things 'donor conception'. My eternal gratitude also goes out to those who provided their feedback on specific sections of this book: to Matty Wright and Terry Masson for your input on transgender individuals; to the wonderful group of transracial donor-conceived people who took the time to get together to discuss and dissect (oh, so gently and kindly) my original piece; to Fabián Guido who gave it a final review; to Amy White for your feedback on the donor section; to Emma-Lee Still for your input on DNA testing; to my beautiful sister Diane McArthur for your feedback on pretty much everything and to my beautiful friend Louise Wigg for sharing your knowledge and wisdom around weight and size-inclusivity.

A heartfelt thanks to Courtney du Toit, who not only provided the most incredibly detailed legal review, but also threw in her first-rate humour for free. I am also grateful (and, I confess, a little sad) that there is much of this book you will never see thanks to Courtney: 'Um, I like what you've written Gail, but I *must* advise you to delete that!'

A very special thank you to my wonderful friend and web developer, Susan Whiteford for helping me with my website, and to Jacinta Calabro for your inspiration and guidance around all things social media.

To my beautiful friends for their ongoing faith and unflagging support over the last decade and for repeatedly asking: 'Are you done yet?' (Yes, I *really* am.) Thank you to Louise Wigg, Michelle Conder, Raechel Thomson, Eiley Ormsby, Jacinta Calabro, Michelle Borg, Nicholas de Castella, Susan Whiteford, Theresa Malin, Caroline Medcraft, Emma Hodgson; to the wise and beautiful women in my women's circle; and, of course, to you Mum—there aren't enough words to describe how incredible you are.

To my editor, my deepest appreciation for your valuable feedback, your remarkable attention to detail and your unfailing kindness; I can't imagine a better partner in this process.

Most of all, thank you to my beautiful daughter for putting up with me for ten years while I wrote this book about donor conception. Your wisdom constantly astounds me, your ability to speak up for what you want is both painful yet promising for your future, and your endless supply of love lifts me up. I love and adore you.

Finally, I'd like to thank you, my readers. I hope you find the information in this book as useful as I know I would have more than a decade ago—and may your children reap the benefits.

Gail Pascoe

Note

The quotes in this book have been generously provided, with permission, by individuals via interview, social media, personal conversations or in response to a direct request from the author. Unless otherwise stated after the quote, individuals have chosen to remain anonymous to protect their privacy.

The opinions expressed in this book do not represent all donor-conceived voices.

Glossary of Acronyms

AI	artificial insemination
ANZICA	Australian and New Zealand Infertility Counsellors Association
ART	assisted reproductive technology
BIPOC	Black, Indigenous (and) People of Colour
FET	frozen embryo transfer
FS	fertility specialist
FSANZ	Fertility Society of Australia and New Zealand
GP	general practitioner
ICI	intracervical insemination
ICSI	intracytoplasmic sperm injection
IP	intended parent
IUI	intrauterine insemination
IVI	intravaginal insemination
IVF	in vitro fertilisation
NHMRC	National Health and Medical Research Council
NI	natural insemination (insemination by penile–vaginal penetration or sexual intercourse)
LGBTQIA+	lesbian, gay, bisexual, transgender, queer/questioning, intersex, asexual and other sexually or gender diverse people
POC	Person of Colour (or People of Colour)
RP	recipient parent
RTAC	Reproductive Technology Accreditation Committee
SMC	solo-mum-by-choice
SPC	solo-parent-by-choice
VARTA	Victorian Assisted Reproductive Treatment Authority

Introduction

We lie in bed together and she rests on one elbow looking directly at me.

'You didn't want to come out,' I explain. 'So, the doctor had to help.'

'And then what happened?' she asks, wide-eyed, lying on her three-year-old belly looking up at me. I have her full attention.

'Well, then he helped you to come out and handed you up to me.' I am transported back to the birthing room. I smile at the memory. 'Then I held you in my arms and said, "Hello! I've been looking forward to meeting you."'

'Oh!' she says with a beautiful smile, her eyes lit up. 'Did you really say that?'

'Yes, I did.'

'And did my donor hold me too?'

'Oh!' This takes me by surprise. My heart breaks a little.

'No,' I respond gently. 'He wasn't there. He lives in America, which is a very long way away. But maybe you can meet him one day?' I hope.

Probably shouldn't have said that . . .

'Yes! I want to meet him one day,' she says, eyes gleaming.

I backpedal, trying to undo my earlier statement. 'I can't make any promises but, maybe, one day you might. And if you don't get to meet him, you can definitely meet lots of your brothers and sisters.' This, I *can* promise. 'Would you like that?'

'Yes! Yes!' She says excitedly. Then a frown. Mulls it over. 'Just my sisters, I think. I don't like boys.'

My own experience

When I skipped eagerly past the exquisite Hybrid Tea roses at the front door of my Canberra fertility clinic thirteen years ago, aged forty-two, preparing to receive an embryo created with a perfect stranger, I thought I had all the answers.

The truth is I had a few answers, but the problem was I didn't know all of the *questions* and, more importantly, I'd asked the questions of the *wrong people*. I'd rebuffed the offer of sperm from several friends: one who'd separated from his wife two weeks earlier; another who lived a thousand kilometres away; and another who hadn't really asked permission from his wife. What followed, before I'd even bent down to smell said roses, was a directive from my chosen clinic to login to their affiliated US sperm bank's website and choose from a catalogue of several dozen available donors.

'This is your best option', they said. 'We don't have any local donors'—so, I complied. Three IVF cycles and one miscarriage later, I gave birth to my beautiful daughter.

Once I'd overcome the initial shock of becoming a parent (I don't think you really quite *get* it until they arrive, no matter how much people warn you), I started to wonder whether Lola[2] had any siblings. Given my donor is American and I used a clinic in Georgia, I thought it likely she had a handful of siblings scattered across the USA and perhaps even up to Canada—but what about Australia? Was there a sister living down the road; twins in the Barossa; a brother in Port Douglas?

I decided to investigate . . . and promptly fell off my breastfeeding rocker. *Thirty-five* siblings! I sat motionless for quite some time, my mouth forming a perfect 'O'. I wondered what those children looked like. Did they have blonde hair, or black? Green eyes, or brown? What were their parents like? Would we like each other and, you know, hang out?

And the big question: Should I make contact?

Of course, the answer was a resounding 'Yes' and today I know that my daughter has in excess of one hundred siblings. Sadly, no one will ever know the exact number, not even the sperm bank that helped create her.

Be informed

Assisted reproductive technology (ART) is a controversial topic for many and evokes a range of responses triggered by factors such as religion, culture, politics, ethics and science. Some people believe ART should be available to anyone who wants it, while others find it ethically problematic, claiming people are placing their own needs above those of their children. Others believe ART is tampering with nature.[3] Placing a donor into the mix only adds to the controversy, *especially* for the donor-conceived people born as a result.

Whatever your opinion, donor conception is here to stay and for many (myself included) using a donor offers the only possible means of building a family. In fact, the number of people undergoing donor conception in Australia has increased so much that many clinics claim the majority of their clientele are solo parents and LGBTQIA+ families who access ART treatment using a donor.

Hollywood appears to have been on trend for decades, having produced a string of movies and television series addressing the topic with varying degrees of integrity and awareness (mostly at the lower end). These movies include, but are not limited to, *Made in America* (1993), *21 Grams* (2003), *The Back-up Plan* (2010), *Delivery Man* (2013), *Almost Family* (2019–20) and *The Sex Lives of College Girls* (premiered 2021).

Australia jumped on the bandwagon in 2017 with the series, *Sisters,* about a woman whose father, a fertility specialist, makes a death bed confession to his daughter that he used his own sperm to impregnate unsuspecting patients and the possibility that she may have hundreds of siblings. Is this scenario even possible, or is it just small-screen nonsense?

While I have no regrets, there is absolutely no question that I dived headfirst into the murky waters of donor conception without checking the depth. After all, I wanted to have a baby and, at forty, my few remaining eggs were only just managing dog paddle. (You're right: eggs don't really swim; they are transported—but you get the gist.)

So how does one go about conceiving a child using another person's gametes or embryos?

If you've done some research already, you will have discovered there is information aplenty 'out there', but it is all distinctly compartmentalised. Everything you want (and need) to know requires an exhaustive amount of time and effort frequenting multiple social media sites, a variety of news media and numerous clinic websites. Sometimes, the information you find is confusing, misleading and, on occasion, untrue.

Even so, is there *really* enough information out there to fully inform people and help them make critical decisions that will have lifelong repercussions for parents, donors and, more importantly, donor-conceived people? For instance, a large proportion of articles written about donor conception are overtly parent-centred and make little or no mention of the impact on the children conceived by this method. When I discovered my daughter had over one hundred siblings, I started doing some digging and, while I found many, many heart-warming stories, a lot of what I uncovered appalled me.

That was ten years ago.

Today, after countless hours of research, including speaking with literally hundreds of people from the donor conception triad (donor-conceived people, donors and recipient parents); fertility specialists and staff at both Australian and international clinics, agencies and egg and sperm banks; fertility counsellors; family lawyers; researchers; authors and more, my initial frame of reference regarding donor conception—which can only be described as breathtaking ignorance—has shifted so remarkably that I feel compelled to share my findings with anyone who will listen.

What are the risks involved in donor conception? Should you choose an Australian donor who doesn't get paid, or should you contribute to an American student's college tuition fees? Should you travel to another country and select a donor who comes with the status 'anonymous'? What if you can't afford a fertility clinic: is it safe to use a stranger sourced from a social media matching site or accept the offer of a neighbour from across the street? What are the repercussions for your donor-conceived children when they discover they have one hundred siblings, or that their 'ID Release at eighteen' donor doesn't actually want anything to do with them. . . ever?

My intentions

> *When we share our stories, donor-conceived people are often told that our experiences are not representative and that 'not all' donor-conceived people feel the way we feel. But this is an obstacle to productive conversation. It is a hindrance to improvement. It is denying an entire group of people their lived reality. It is dismissing the experience of that same group and it works to sweep under the rug the problems with donor conception. We need to replace 'not all' with 'one is too many'. If any amount of people are being harmed by donor conception, then the way donor conception is done needs to be re-examined. Our stories matter and shouldn't be dismissed just because there are some people who haven't suffered as much.*
>
> **American donor-conceived adult**

Let's get the #notalldonorconceivedpeople disclaimer out of the way sooner rather than later. The industry narrative tells us that, as long as our donor-conceived children are told about their conception status, they will be okay. This is true for many, but not for all donor-conceived people.

While this book presents many wonderful stories, it also exposes another side of the donor conception experience and some of the information may shock you (or maybe it won't). This book highlights much that is wrong with the industry, including unethical elements that exist within the culture of donor conception, and it calls attention to the harm that is still, to this day, being done to donor-conceived people. It shines a bright light on the stories that *need* to be told.

You may be wondering at this point whether it is my intention to turn you off the notion of donor conception and to present you with a picture that describes only 'doom and gloom'. The answer to that question is *absolutely not*. There are many wonderful success stories in the world of donor conception and, of course, many of us need assistance from a donor to help build our families. My true goal is to arm you with all of the necessary information; presented from all the perspectives so that you can make informed, calculated decisions and identify and reject unethical practices that may bring harm to your child. I want to help you avoid the mistakes of well-meaning people who have gone before you (myself included).

Ultimately, it is my goal that you, personally, will be instrumental in driving much-needed change to an industry that desperately needs it, so that you and, more importantly, your donor-conceived children can be a success story.

About this book

The questions that surround the decision to use a donor are many and complex. The 'how to?' is even more complex. This book takes a new approach to answering all of these questions and more. It is a step-by-step guide for people who wish to pursue their dream of having children but need assistance from a donor to do so.

The book brings together all of the information you need and presents it in one place. It explains every aspect of the process, including the options available, suggestions regarding how to select a donor, the pros and cons of choosing a local versus international donor, how to find your children's siblings, the needs of donor-conceived people and much, much more. The book is full of real-life stories and quotes from people who have been a part of the donor conception journey you may now be considering.

There are eight distinct parts to the book so, depending on where you are on your personal journey, you may wish to read the book from start to finish, chapter by chapter; or skip parts that don't apply right now and come back to them later. Some parts may not apply to you at all.

People reading from a different perspective (for example, donors, partners or parents of donors, health professionals, or others) may wish to proceed directly to topics that apply to their own individual circumstances.

As parents and potential parents, know that your donor-conceived child will have unique needs and the path you select is worthy of your deep consideration and exploration. Furthermore, many of the topics in this book intersect, so having a broad understanding of the different scenarios and perspectives will help you to make more informed decisions moving forward.

I am so grateful to be able to present the information in this book which I believe will benefit you and, even more importantly, your donor-conceived child.

This is the book I needed to read when I was making my decision. I hope you enjoy it and I wish you every success with building your family.

Gail Pascoe

Conscious conception

> *. . . Look and listen for the welfare of the whole people and have always in view not only the present but also the coming generations, even those whose faces are yet beneath the surface of the ground—the unborn of the future Nation.*
>
> **Excerpt from the Constitution of the Iroquois Nations**[4]

All cultures are rich with their own versions of wisdom and intelligence; knowledge and insights gathered through the passage of time and experience. For instance, the Iroquois, a First Nations people of North America, live by a philosophy called the 'Seventh Generation Principle'. This means that, for every proposed act of change, the leaders determine how the change might impact the next seven generations. What incredible wisdom.

Sadly, this kind of philosophy and foresight has been missing from the process of donor conception and, while Australia is certainly ahead of the game compared to many other countries and there is definitely some activity in Australia to support our donor-conceived children, little time or energy has been given to understanding what the future holds for generations of donor-conceived people. Will they each wear a necklace with the donor's ID clearly visible, or have it tattooed on their body? Will potential partners need to send saliva off to a laboratory for DNA testing to ensure they are not about to enter into a sexual relationship with a sibling? Will there be people trawling the internet looking for donors and siblings, trying to find the missing pieces of their fractured jigsaw puzzle? Will those same people be denigrated and shamed on social media for expressing a desire to look for their biological parents? Will they be told they are being disrespectful, selfish and ungrateful?

The truth is, all of these things are already happening.

And what of the teenagers, the 'tweens', or the babes in arms? What of the new generations of donor-conceived people who have known their conception status from birth and are free to discuss issues as they arise with their fully-informed and self-aware parents? Are they 'owning' and loving their conception status? Are the problems cited by previous generations of people now obsolete tropes? Or are we, in some instances, repeating patterns from the past—for example, choosing anonymous foreign donors; or telling children their conception status too late, if at all? Is it conceivable that we might be creating *new* problems, such as the impact on children who discover that the teenage egg donor who assisted with their creation was exploited with the promise of a new car (and has the TikTok video to prove it); or the language and cultural barriers resulting from the selection of donors who reside on the other side of the globe; or the impact on children who find themselves with hundreds of siblings?

In any event, how will our children fare as they move into adulthood?

There's no question that, around the world right now, the dialogue surrounding donor conception is intensifying. Unethical industry practices are being called out, laws are being changed and new ones are being introduced.

So, what can you do to help the next seven generations of donor-conceived people? The biggest impact you can have is to start your parenting journey with the intention of 'conscious conception'. This means making sure that you, your partner (if you have one), and your donor(s) are mentally, emotionally, physically and spiritually ready to bring a new person into the world; that your body is as healthy as it possibly can be; and that your heart and mind are open. It means educating yourself about the possibilities and the implications of donor conception, as well as making informed choices to support your child's wellbeing.

It also means recognising whether your donor (and their partner and family, if possible) fully understand the implications of what they are offering and that you consider at length, whether they are the right donor for you.

You also need to imagine a future with your donor-conceived child—a little human being who will later become an independent, thinking, feeling adult—and ask yourself whether you will be able to openly share the details of their conception with them, guide them through any feelings and emotions they may have about their origins, and lead and support them with love and an open heart in attempts to connect with their siblings and biological parent(s). It means accepting the possibility that, despite your feelings of deep and unconditional love for your child, there are no guarantees they will not experience 'negative' feelings and emotions related to various aspects of their conception story.

If we take a deliberate and conscious approach to conception, we can learn from the previous generations of donor-conceived people and, together, we can offer our children the best possible start in life, easing them on their way into a happy and healthy future.

Part One: Getting Started

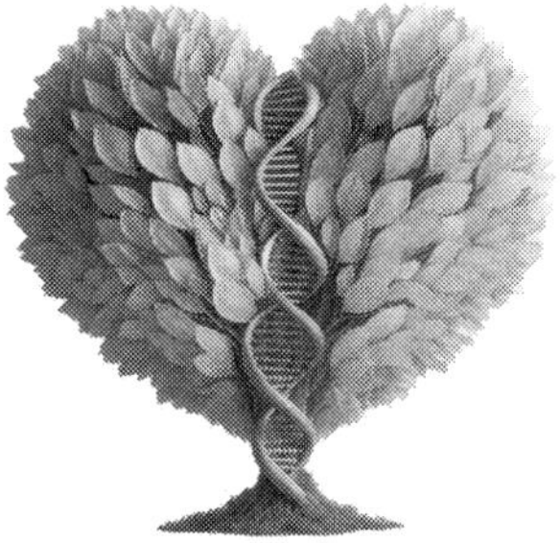

As a donor-conceived person, my advice to anyone considering donor conception would be to do as much research as you can before starting out. Make sure you and your partner, if you have one, are emotionally ready to do this; educate yourself on industry practices that are unethical; talk to lots and lots of donor-conceived people so you can understand their perspectives and be aware that your donor-conceived child will have specific needs that other children don't have. And take your time!

Australian donor-conceived adult (Vic.)

Using a donor to build your family is a process filled with complexities and nuances and, indeed, the internet does not provide all of the answers. Where to get started? What to do first? Who to talk to?

The next three chapters provide some background about donor conception, why people undertake it and the things you need to know if you or your partner are not going to be biologically related to your child.

1

What is Donor Conception?

Donor conception is the process of having a baby using donated sperm, eggs or embryos through self-insemination or fertility treatment such as IVF.

The Victorian Assisted Reproductive Treatment Authority[5]

Donation of gametes (sperm and eggs) and embryos is the act of giving one's gametes to another person with the intention of assisting that person to conceive a child. And while the term 'donor' applies in Australia where all donations must be altruistic, it becomes an imprecise term when describing people who receive payment for their gametes. 'Gamete provider', is an oft-used term to cover this anomaly. Some donor-conceived people even feel uncomfortable about small reimbursements having been paid to the donor.

Around the world, including in Australia, the practice of non-disclosure of their conception stories to children has been so prolific, and subsequent data collection so inaccurate, that there is no way of knowing how many donor-conceived people exist today.[6] While more research is being done, the number of studies related to donor conception are limited, they are frequently biased towards participants who self-select (that is, people who already know they are donor conceived and are intrinsically motivated to participate) and many studies are heavily skewed toward female participants.

Most sperm and egg donors proactively harvest their gametes with the express purpose of allowing another person to use them. Embryo donation, which occurs less frequently, is different altogether and usually arises as a result of a person or couple undergoing assisted reproductive treatment (ART) to conceive their own child and embryos being left over afterwards. Some international embryo agencies also intentionally create embryos from donor gametes using their own pre-screened sperm and egg donors.

Embryo donation is unique in that children born from embryos can have full genetic siblings from the donating parents—and in some cases, if the donating parents used a donor, there can be half-siblings as well. (For more information about embryo donation see Chapter 9, 'Choosing Your Donor[s]'.)

Double donation describes the process whereby the recipient requires both an egg donor and a sperm donor. Individually selected donor eggs and sperm, sometimes from different countries, are used to create embryos which are then made available to the recipient(s). Double donation is different from embryo donation because the two donors are chosen separately by the intended parent, whereas embryo donation arises when excess embryos have been created by an existing couple (including donor gametes in some instances), or by an embryo agency/clinic.

2

Why People Use Donor Gametes and Embryos

The number of people using sperm, egg and embryo donors to conceive has increased dramatically and continues to increase. So why are people pursuing these options?

People with medical infertility or inheritable disorders, single parents, and many LGBTQIA+ singles, couples and people in multi-partner relationships, may require a donor to create their families.

Medical infertility is experienced by one in six Australian couples and this problem is shared equally between sexes. The fertility of men and people who produce sperm can be impacted by many things including: a sporting injury; radiotherapy or chemotherapy; a previous vasectomy; or exposure to everyday environmental toxins that can result in a low sperm count. Common causes of infertility in women and people who produce eggs include: irregular ovulation; blockages in the fallopian tubes; abnormalities of the uterus or cervix; disorders such as polycystic ovary syndrome and endometriosis;[7] poorly developed or inaccessible ovaries; no ovaries; poor egg quality; and early menopause.

There are also multiple reasons that some single people use donors with the intention of parenting a child on their own. This demographic, known as 'solo mums by choice' (SMC) or 'solo parents by choice' (SPC), now makes up the vast majority of people seeking donor sperm.[8] For instance, people in this situation often use a donor because they have not yet met a partner with whom they wish to conceive, or they have left relationships to find themselves suddenly single and childless. In other instances, people may have a history of relationship trauma, or sexual (or other) abuse, making the option of having a partner an undesirable proposition at the time.

Depending on their individual circumstances and relationships, many LGBTQIA+ individuals, couples and multi-partnered people require the assistance of a donor.

3

Being the Non-biological Parent

. . . a genetic connection is not required for the parent-child attachment process to occur because of the nature of attachment. Think about the people you love whom you are not related to—like your spouse or partner. A loving attachment happens when you spend time with someone every day.[9]

Jana M. Rupnow (author of *Three Makes Baby*)

> ***Note:*** The term, 'biological parent', is used in this book to identify people who are *genetically* related to their child. To avoid confusion, people who carry and give birth to a child, but are not genetically related to that child, are referred to as 'gestational parents'. The author does acknowledge that carrying a child is a biological process encompassing more than just genetics and that the term 'biological mother/parent' is also widely used by people who have used egg donors.

Many people find themselves parenting a child to whom they are not genetically related. At one end of the spectrum this scenario does not present any issues at all but, for others, being biologically unrelated to their child can be deeply distressing and frightening.

For those experiencing medical infertility, social media abounds with dialogue about the journeys of others who have experienced failed pregnancy tests; miscarriages; loss of self-esteem; being told to 'just relax and it will happen'; being asked whether adoption has been considered; and the pain of being invited to others' baby showers—tens of thousands of people finding solace in a shared grief online.

Feelings of loss can be overwhelming and compounding. For instance, you may feel a loss of control; financial loss; loss of hope; loss of emotional stability; grief for the loss of a pregnancy in the case of a miscarriage; and much, much more. When combined, it can feel like these losses are a threat to your survival—a life crisis. Depending on your circumstances, you may not be willing—or able—to share your grief with family and friends. Sometimes, the people around you simply don't understand your grief.[10]

While research indicates that the absence of a genetic connection between young children and their parents does not necessarily risk the development of a positive relationship,[11] it could create obstacles if personal issues, related to infertility or otherwise, have not been worked through. Some examples might include difficulty bonding with the child, wondering whether the child will love you, feeling jealous of a partner who does have a genetic connection to the child, shame and embarrassment related to not being a 'legitimate' parent, disappointment that the child does not look like you, or fear that the child will 'run off' with the donor.

Sometimes being genetically unrelated to a child prompts people to lie to their child about their conception, but it's important to know that when a secret of this magnitude is unveiled (frequently through direct-to-consumer DNA testing) the costs of secrecy can be high and, in some cases, catastrophic (see Chapter 14, 'Talking about Donor Conception').

Before starting the process of donor conception, it is vital to address any of the feelings that could arise from being a non-biological parent. Jana Rupnow, psychotherapist and fertility counsellor, explains:

> *Your new child will be depending on you to show them the way and guide them toward acceptance of their personal life story. Your child will need to feel a sense of belonging in your family while also feeling free to express their differences.*[12]

Making the transition to becoming a non-biological parent is not something to be rushed. Have you given yourself sufficient time to understand and grieve the loss of your fertility (if relevant)? Have you worked through any feelings of anger, sadness, shame, resentment or other emotions similar to these? Do you feel equipped to handle other people's questions about your status as a parent? If you are partnered, have you communicated with each other about the mental, emotional and spiritual implications of being a non-biological parent? Are you comfortable with your partner being the gestational parent (if that is the case)? Do you have a strategy in place to address any ongoing issues that might arise?

> *You can't expect your child to be comfortable being donor-conceived if you are not.*
>
> **Victorian Assisted Reproductive Treatment Authority (VARTA)**[13]

It's important to know that, if you don't work through any issues and you carry the subsequent emotional burdens with you through the process of parenting, you are likely to pass them on to your child which may then present as shame of being donor-conceived. Australian donor-conceived adult, Matty Wright, explains:

> *As a donor-conceived person* [myself], *know that your insecurities around your status as a parent will subtly affect your child's development, so try to sort them out beforehand.*

Sometimes people don't wish to address these concerns until after a child is born, but this may be too late.

Your fertility specialist and team should be addressing the medical aspects of your donor conception journey quite well, but it is not necessarily within their purview to manage your feelings and emotions. If you need help to work through any feelings or issues, it is a good idea to seek assistance from a person qualified in this area—make sure that person is experienced in the nuances of donor conception. In addition, social media support groups exist where people having similar experiences can assist you with working through any issues you may have and may also provide ongoing support.

Part Two:
Donor Types

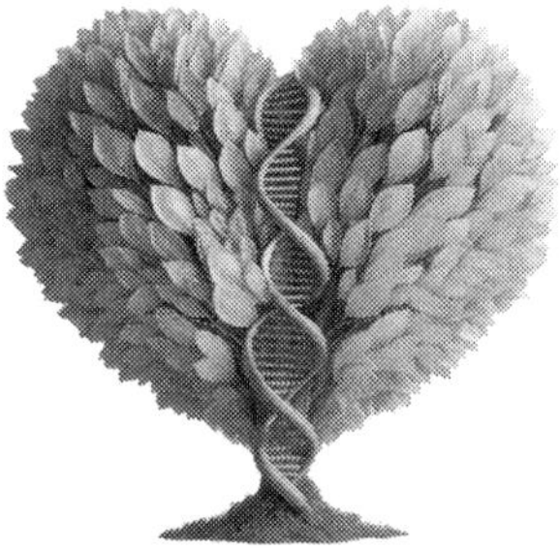

I've seen people choose donors for all sorts of reasons, and often those reasons are about themselves as the parent—what's convenient, cheaper, quicker (and these reasons are pretty triggering to be honest). But people really need to put their future child first when making decisions. They need to start thinking, 'How will the choices I make affect my child, a person who will be an adult for a lot longer than they'll be a child?'

Australian donor-conceived adult

It is important to understand the different donor types, how the related processes work, and the subsequent pros and cons of each process. As is true for most things, the choices you make will have a significant impact on your life and the life of your child.

The next three chapters outline the donor types and, while you may come across various names and titles for donors, for the purposes of this book donors have been classified into the following three categories:

1. clinic-recruited donors (donors recruited by Australian fertility clinics)
2. international donors (donors recruited overseas and whose gametes are imported to Australia; or donors recruited in foreign countries so intended parents travel overseas to receive the donated gametes)
3. known donors (donors known to the intended parent[s])—the extent to which a donor is known to the recipient can vary significantly from case to case.

> ***Note:*** Surrogacy is not dealt with in this book.

If you're not ready to read about different donor types yet, skip this part and come back later, although it may be helpful to understand the basics discussed on the following pages before you move to Part 3, 'Making decisions'.

4

Clinic-recruited Donors

What is a fertility clinic?

Fertility clinics were first established to help heterosexual married couples who had infertility issues have children. Over time, as the definition of 'family' has evolved and single-parent and LGBTQIA+ people have been able to build their families, clinics have adapted to meet the needs of a broader clientele.

Fertility clinics are well-oiled machines that follow strict protocols and adhere to rigid timeframes. They cleverly manage people's reproductive cycles to fit in around optimum timing for egg collection and fertilisation, as well as staff availability and other practical matters. They make no promises about conception (although sometimes they might, and that can be problematic).[14]

What is a clinic-recruited donor?

As the name suggests, these are people who wish to become donors and are recruited by (most) fertility clinics. In all cases, donors are required to meet certain criteria and undergo extensive screening to ensure they are suitable (see Chapter 13, 'Being a Donor and How it Works'). Clinic-recruited donors must also consent to having their identifying details released; a status known as 'ID Release'.

What is identity (ID) release?

> *ID release is really just 'Anonymous Lite'.*
>
> **New Zealand sperm donor**

In Australia, clinic-recruited donors cannot be anonymous and, when they sign up, must consent to having identity (ID) release status.[15]

In other words, donors must agree to their identifying details being accessible to their donor-conceived offspring when they turn a certain age (check with your clinic regarding the rules which apply in that jurisdiction).

From the perspective of donor-conceived people, it is useful to know that many feel the 'ID Release' rule to be akin to a 'bait and switch' scheme (offering a person something desirable to gain favour then thwarting expectations with something less desirable). This attitude arises from the feeling that eighteen years of age (or any other specified age) is too long to wait to connect with one's biological parent—a person who may not even be interested in connecting; whose contact details may be out of date; or, even worse, who may be deceased by the time a child attempts to make contact. Essentially, the ID Release rule makes a donor anonymous for eighteen years (or the time specified).

> *I don't think people really understand the grief involved with not knowing who your biological parent is until eighteen. All that time lost is time you can't get back. Finding your biological parent as an adult is like trying to go home to a home you've never been to.*
>
> **Australian donor-conceived adult (WA)**

My daughter Lola[16] agrees with this sentiment and has expressed that, 'ID Release is a stupid rule and eighteen years is a lifetime.'

Interestingly, some countries around the world are lowering this age and, in Germany, as long as it can be proven that the child makes the request for information to know their biological parent, there is no minimum age.[17]

Types of donors

Sperm donors

In the case of clinic-recruited sperm donors, people attend the clinic for an agreed period of time to provide semen samples (see Chapter 13, 'Being a Donor and How it Works'). The clinics then make the sperm available to people who wish to conceive via assisted reproductive technology (ART) (see Chapter 11, 'Assisted Reproductive Technology [ART], "At-home" Insemination, Success Rates and Costs'). On rare occasions, it is also possible that a person may wish to donate leftover frozen sperm after having undergone ART treatment with their own partner.

Egg donors

Clinic-recruited egg donors become available: when an individual specifically elects to undergo a stimulation cycle at a clinic with the sole intention of donating their eggs; when someone who previously elected to freeze their eggs might no longer require them; or when a person who has completed one or more IVF cycles might have no use for their remaining frozen eggs (although, in most cases, a person would attempt to fertilise all of their eggs after retrieval and would only have remaining embryos).

Embryo donors

Clinic-recruited embryos become available when a person (or couple) completes their ART treatment and the decision is made by them to donate their excess embryos; the embryos might have been created from their own gametes or from donor gametes.

Why clinic-recruited donors are in short supply

The number of clinic-recruited sperm donors has decreased slightly in the past few years, but there is also an increase in demand.[18] And while the number of clinic-recruited sperm donors is often low (or is occasionally zero at some clinics), the frequency of people putting up their hands to be clinic-recruited *egg* donors is even more limited, resulting in the recipients' waiting period being so long that some clinics don't even bother with this option.

Some people believe that Australian clinics should direct some of their spectacularly large income streams into the donor-recruitment process, but it appears they don't do so because recruiting, screening and maintaining a donor pool is expensive—and probably doesn't make them too much money. It would seem that telling people, 'Go find your own donor, then come back and see us,' or encouraging the use of international gametes via their affiliated sperm or egg bank, requires significantly less effort for some providers.

The shortage of clinic-recruited donors in Australia is due to a combination of factors, including:

- the commitment required (for example, sperm donors are required to attend a clinic multiple times, often for several months)
- the lack of financial incentives for those who wish to be paid for their donation
- concerns about the short-term and long-term health risks of donating eggs
- fears about a lack of control over selection of recipients and, as a result of that, choosing to become a known donor instead
- concerns about whether the recipient parents would agree to early contact or not, including subsequent concerns regarding the safety and wellbeing of their biological child
- for many people, donating can feel like they are 'giving away' their own prospective children.

Why people use clinic-recruited donors

Sperm donors

While ART treatment at a clinic is expensive, one of the primary reasons people use a clinic-recruited sperm donor is to maximise their own safety and that of their child. Measures of that safety include the reduced risk of STIs and inherited diseases, and the fact that donors are required to sign documents indicating they do not have an intention to claim parenting rights (see Chapter 16, 'ART Regulations and Ethical Guidelines').

Another reason people use clinic-recruited donors is due to fertility issues and a clinic can potentially increase the chances of conception. People who have had unsatisfactory experiences with finding a known sperm donor or feel daunted by the process (see Chapter 6, 'Known Donors') may also turn to a clinic-recruited donor as a better option.

> **Note:** It's important to understand that, despite the perceived safety, there are still multiple risks involved in undergoing ART treatment with a donor at an Australian clinic (see Chapter 11, 'Assisted Reproductive Technology [ART], "At-home" Insemination, Success Rates and Costs').

Egg donors

The process for using donated eggs is significantly more complex than the process for using donated sperm. If a clinic has its own egg donors available, an enormous amount of time and effort can be saved for intended parents who would otherwise be required to find their own donors.

Conception

If you choose to conceive with a clinic-recruited sperm or egg donor, you will be required to participate in some form of ART treatment. The type of treatment you undergo will depend on a multitude of factors, such as your age, fertility, availability of treatments at your chosen clinic, your reproductive history, and more (see Chapter 11, 'Assisted Reproductive Technology [ART], "At-home" Insemination, Success Rates and Costs').

How does it work?

At the risk of stating the obvious, the anatomical constructs for producing sperm and eggs are quite different. As a result of this distinction, it is *significantly* easier, less time-consuming, less invasive and much safer from a health perspective, for people to donate sperm than it is for people to donate eggs. This fact has many implications for donor conception, one of these being that there are generally fewer egg donors available than there are sperm donors. Another implication is that the fertility of women and people who produce eggs begins to decline earlier than does the fertility of men and people who produce sperm, so the upper age limits for egg donors are much lower than those for sperm donors. Egg donors are unable to donate when they are pregnant or breastfeeding and this also reduces the time for which they are available to donate. Furthermore, the number of children a person can create via their egg donations is considerably less than the number someone can create via sperm donations (although there are cases overseas where egg donors have produced large numbers of children).

In all cases when donor eggs are used, both the egg donor and the recipient are required to undergo ART treatment.

It is also interesting to note that the fertility industry tends to treat egg donation and sperm donation quite differently. Rene Almeling highlights multiple differences in her book, *Sex cells: The medical market for eggs and sperm,* and notes that the divergence between the approaches begins at the clinic or bank level where interactions between donors and staff take place:

> *Drawing on cultural ideals of maternal femininity and paternal masculinity, staff frame egg donation as a gift and sperm donation as a job.*[19]

The donor treatment process for intended parents

All clinics have a process similar to the one described on the following pages (but the process, and the order in which it occurs, can vary between clinics).

> ***Note:*** Depending on where you live, if you are using public sperm and egg bank services, you may be required to attend multiple appointments *locally* at a partner centre, and then to attend the appropriate facility to undergo the ART treatment itself—for example IVF (see Chapter 11, 'Assisted Reproductive Technology [ART], "At-home" Insemination, Success Rates and Costs').

Referral

You need a referral from your health professional to ensure that you (and your partner, if that applies) are eligible for Medicare rebates for consultations and treatments. If you are not eligible for Medicare rebates, this will result in *significantly* higher costs for fertility treatment (see Chapter 11, 'Assisted Reproductive Technology [ART], "At-home" Insemination, Success Rates and Conceiving Costs').

Appointment with a fertility specialist

Once you have obtained a referral, you (and your partner, if applicable) can make an appointment with a fertility specialist who will collect information and discuss matters related to your personal circumstances (such as medical conditions, menstrual history and pregnancy history), in order to determine the appropriate treatment for you. You may be advised to undergo various diagnostic testing procedures to ensure that fertility treatment using donor gametes is a suitable option for you.

The specialist will provide you with a list of pre-pregnancy tests to complete, which may include tests for such things as HIV, chlamydia and Rubella; your blood group, Rh factor, and iron levels; and some tests relating to ovulation and other aspects of fertility. Testing is usually completed at your own expense but, in some cases, it may be bulk-billed.

Note: Depending on the clinic, or if you are using public sperm and egg bank services, you may be required to undergo all of the testing procedures before you attend an appointment with the fertility specialist (see Chapter 7, 'Choosing an Australian Fertility Clinic').

Counselling and information sessions

It is a requirement for recipients of donor gametes (and their partners, if applicable) to attend counselling prior to completing a fertility treatment. Some clinics expect you to attend more than one session and, if your donor is known to you or you are undergoing embryo donation, a group session may be required. Check with your clinic regarding the rules which apply in that jurisdiction.

Counselling provides the opportunity to discuss any concerns or fears you may have about using a donor and should better prepare you to address the needs of your donor-conceived child.

In the counselling session, the counsellor should discuss topics including, but not limited to, the potential long-term psychosocial implications for families and children born as a result of donor conception; the rights and responsibilities of all parties related to information disclosure; and the support available to you.[20] You might also discuss the mental, emotional and physical demands of fertility treatment, how many cycles you might be willing to complete and how you will cope if the treatment is unsuccessful.

If there is a lengthy waiting period (for example, many months or even years) between applying for gametes or embryos and subsequently becoming eligible, you may be required to undergo further counselling to ensure you receive up-to-date information regarding processes or legislation and to check you have not changed your mind.

Unfortunately, it appears that the quality of counselling can vary significantly from clinic to clinic. The counselling can also be severely lacking in discourse concerning the potential issues we now understand can be experienced by donor-conceived people as they grow and, therefore, the potential challenges the parent(s) might face raising a donor-conceived child. Some parents reported a positive experience:

> *We had several counselling sessions, including one with my egg donor, and the counsellor was excellent. She was pragmatic, had a lot of empathy and was also assertive about discussing uncomfortable topics.*

But others describe a vastly different experience:

> *The counsellor was very impersonal. She asked me why I wanted to use a donor, went through the legalities, asked me to sign the form and said thank you. It felt like a tick-the-box exercise.*

This parent went on to say, 'I could've done a better job myself,' and that sentiment was echoed by the findings of a 2019 inquiry by the Health Complaints Commissioner into Victorian ART practices,[21] which found that: counselling was often seen by patients as a 'tick-the-box' exercise; some people were frightened to ask questions in case they were denied treatment; counsellors were hard to access during treatment cycles; and doubts were expressed as to whether counsellors are adequately trained to assist people undergoing ART treatment.

If possible, find a counsellor you trust, prepare yourself with a list of questions and then provide feedback (or make a complaint) if you feel a counselling session did not meet your needs.

Cooling-off period

Chances are you didn't just wake up this morning and decide: 'I'm going to give this baby thing a go and find myself a donor.' Even if you did, using a donor is an option that needs to be considered at length. It is a topic you need to test out with family, friends and your partner (if you have one); and warrants being investigated with quite a bit of Googling. The cooling-off period is time in which you are allowed to change your mind; check with your clinic regarding the duration of their cooling-off period, if one applies. Depending on your state or territory, or the individual clinic, this could be a period of several months.

Specialist review or appointment with a nurse

Once you have completed all of your tests, the fertility specialist will recommend a treatment plan. You will then attend another appointment at which the person will take you through the details of the treatment plan (including a general timeline), provide you with any relevant medication and discuss the communication process that will take place during the treatment cycle.

Appointment with a patient liaison administrator

A patient liaison administrator will explain the administrative processes, such as costs and payment methods, and will schedule your appointments with your specialist, counsellor, nurses, and so on. You will be required to sign a form indicating that you are responsible for providing information to the clinic about the outcome of the treatment cycle (for example, a miscarriage or a live birth).[22] This supports accurate data collection and also protects the rights of donor-conceived people by ensuring they have knowledge about how they were conceived.

Choosing your donor

See Chapter 9, 'Choosing Your Donor[s]', and Chapter 11, 'Assisted Reproductive Technology [ART], "At-home" Insemination, Success Rates and Costs'.

If you are bringing your known donor to the clinic to undergo ART treatment, the donor will also be required to attend an appointment with the specialist, undergo counselling, and participate in various other parts of the process. (For more information about known donors, see Chapter 6, 'Known Donors'.)

Treatment

Once you have undergone all of the requisite steps and the clinic has staff (and donor) availability, your ART treatment will commence using your donor's gametes. Whatever your treatment plan, the clinic will provide you with a detailed schedule outlining the various steps in the process, including appointments and times, blood tests, ultrasounds, and required pharmaceuticals and their respective doses and timing schedules.

All parties involved in the use of donor gametes via a clinic are required to provide valid consent before treatment commences. The consent process is ongoing and not just a single event. This applies to the person undergoing treatment, their partner (if one is involved) and the donor.[23]

5
International Donors

An international donor is someone who donates their gametes in a country overseas. If an Australian clinic has a service agreement with an international sperm or egg bank, frozen gametes can be imported directly to that Australian clinic. Alternatively, some people travel to various foreign countries to undergo ART treatment. As the popularity of these options gains momentum, more and more countries are being added to the mix. However, it is important to note that, while this alternative definitely provides access to more donors, using an international donor comes with its own set of risks and issues, for you *and* for your child.

'Identity (ID) Release' and international donors

> *It's absolutely harder to form connections with genetic family as an adult than it is as a child. I will never understand 'anonymous until eighteen' arrangements. It's absolute crap; not in the best interest of donor-conceived children at all.*
>
> **American donor-conceived adult**

If you use an international donor via an Australian clinic, the ID Release rule also applies (see Chapter 4, 'Clinic-recruited Donors'). However, if you travel overseas to undergo ART treatment, it's important to be aware that terms and definitions can vary from country to country, as well as from bank to bank. Alternative international naming conventions you may see on overseas bank and agency websites include 'open ID', 'open donor', 'ID consenting', 'ID disclosure', 'non-anonymous', and other variants. Never assume these terms equate to the Australian version of ID Release.

For instance, 'open donor' at some international banks means they will try to contact the donor on your behalf when your child turns eighteen but, if the donor fails to respond or changes their mind about contact, they will not release the donor's details to your child. Others define 'open donor' as a facilitated contact between the donor and their donor-conceived child/adult, in some cases without the donor-conceived person actually learning the identity of their biological parent. (Nope, doesn't seem particularly open to me either.) Others explain that their 'open donors' will allow your child a minimum one-time contact when they turn eighteen (which it appears, cannot be guaranteed).

If you are undertaking the travel route to use donor gametes overseas, make sure you do your homework regarding the terms and definitions used *and* the corresponding actuality.

Some donors have reported that they chose Open ID because it pays more, despite them having no intention of being available for contact when their offspring turn the required age.

If you use an international donor via an Australian clinic, your donor's identifying information arrives with the gametes and will be retained at your clinic. If you travelled overseas to use an international donor, your overseas clinic will (hopefully) also retain this data.

While some sperm/egg banks claim to contact their donors on a regular basis for updated information, it's also important to know that many international donors report that, once they've donated, they never hear from the bank or agency again. Some donors even report that they get the cold shoulder when they try to make contact.

This may have implications for your child when they attempt to connect with the donor.

Sperm/egg banks and egg/embryo agencies

> *Some journalists refer to the US fertility industry as 'The Wild West'. I told them that expression makes it sound fun and exciting. I prefer 'clusterfuck'.*
>
> **Erin Jackson (founder of We Are Donor Conceived)**

Sperm banks

Sperm banks, sometimes known as cryobanks (the prefix 'cryo', derived from the Ancient Greek meaning cold or frost), are businesses that collect human sperm from donors and store them for a contracted period of time, in order to assist people who need donor sperm to conceive a child. Sperm banks generally operate independently of clinics and sell their 'product' to whoever wants it. The first sperm banks were established in the 1970s, a couple of decades after it was discovered that human sperm could be frozen and thawed successfully.

Today, sperm banks are a multi-billion-dollar business worldwide and, while they have helped to create a lot of families that might not have existed otherwise, they are considered by some to be complicit in the commodification of children.

Egg banks

While it has been known for a few decades that human eggs could be frozen, the old slow-cooling method did not have high success rates. With the introduction of rapid freezing, called 'vitrification', the use of chemicals known as cryoprotectants prevents water molecules from forming intracellular ice crystals and thereby protects the frozen genetic material. As a result, conception success rates with frozen eggs have improved significantly.

Due to the more complex nature of egg retrieval, there are far fewer egg banks than there are sperm banks and a handful of egg banks tend to dominate the world market.

So, what exactly do egg banks do?

Egg banks are businesses that collect eggs from donors in order to assist people who need donor eggs to conceive a child. In a similar manner to sperm banks, the eggs are frozen and stored, then shipped around the world in cryogenic containers to the recipient's clinic of choice. In some cases, eggs are fertilised with donor sperm first and then shipped as frozen embryos.

Egg banks usually offer guarantees regarding the number of eggs they provide (for example, six or eight), with the option of paying for additional eggs. Their guarantees may also allow for subsequent replacements should the original gametes prove unsuccessful for creating embryos. For example, if six eggs were supplied and they do not result in at least one embryo, recipients might receive a further six eggs for free.

Payments are usually predictable and access to the eggs is simple and convenient because no cycle synchronisation is required between donors and recipients (see Chapter 11, 'Assisted Reproductive Technology [ART], "At-home" Insemination, Success Rates and Costs'). Eggs can be frozen for many years without significant deterioration. Eggs retrieved for freezing from women in their twenties and early thirties generally have higher success rates than those retrieved from older women, so the maximum age requirement for egg donors is usually around thirty-three years of age.

Egg donor agencies

Egg donor agencies recruit donors who can provide the option of undergoing *fresh* embryo transfers (see Chapter 11, 'Assisted Reproductive Technology [ART], "At-home" Insemination, Success Rates and Costs'). Unlike egg banks from which frozen eggs can be accessed at the convenience of the recipient, there are many logistical issues to navigate. These include synchronising donor and recipient menstrual cycles, travel for the recipient and/or the donor, donor availability and the requirement for donor screening prior to each egg retrieval. All of the eggs retrieved during a cycle are received by the intended parent(s) (unless it is a shared cycle), but there is also the possibility of receiving few or no eggs.

Due to all of the logistical considerations involved, using a donor from an egg donor agency may involve a longer waiting period than accessing frozen eggs. Those various considerations can also impact the costs involved (which are usually higher than those for using frozen eggs) and can create unpredictability regarding the calculation of expenses.

Embryo donor agencies/clinics

Donor embryo agencies and clinics are businesses that specialise in providing people with fully-formed embryos. (An egg bank may also offer an option for sourcing embryos.) These agencies and clinics remove the need for a person to select an egg donor and a sperm donor, as well as potentially reducing the extent of ART treatment required (see Chapter 11, 'Assisted Reproductive Technology [ART[, "At-home" Insemination, Success Rates and Costs').

Sometimes international embryo agencies make incredible claims that your donor-conceived child will, through some supernatural manifestation, absorb all of your talents, behaviour and looks simply because you are the gestational parent.[24] Please don't be fooled by these types of claims (see Chapter 9, 'Choosing Your Donor[s]').

It is also important to be aware that, in some countries where local people undergoing IVF have excess embryos in storage, embryos are sometimes given away to people seeking to have a child *without* the owner's permission.[25]

Sometimes embryo agencies proactively create embryos using donor sperm and donor eggs, rather than using unused embryos from people who have undergone IVF cycles. These embryos are often anonymous and fall under a slightly different category again, sometimes referred to as 'double donation embryos', or 'double donor embryos'.

All embryo donations in Australia are from excess embryos following ART treatment.

Why people use international donors

Cross-border reproductive treatment is the process of travelling overseas, or long distances within a particular country, to undergo donor conception.

The terms, 'fertility shopping', 'reproductive tourism' and 'fertility tourism' are also used by some people, however the terms are deemed offensive by many because of the implication that donor-conceived people are a commodity, or the end product of a shopping trip.

Whether undergoing fertility treatment in another country, or remaining in Australia to access imported gametes, there are a number of reasons why people use international donors.

Long waits for local gametes combined, in some instances, with the rapid closure of a person's fertile window may result in the search for more readily available international gametes. Some clinics may have longer wait times for international donors than clinic-recruited donors in cases where only 'exclusive donors' are allowed. (See Chapter 9, 'Choosing Your Donor[s]', for more information regarding 'exclusive donors'.)

International donor profiles also tend to provide much more information, including adult photos, personal essays and audio files, while Australian clinic-recruited donors are frequently limited in number, the personal details provided by them are sparse and they may not meet the intended parents' criteria.

Some people seek a donor from their country of birth who can provide them with children of similar genetic makeup to themselves or, alternatively, genes that reduce the risk of certain diseases.

Sometimes a person may have undergone multiple failed treatments in a local clinic and may believe alternative or superior treatment options are available elsewhere. International gametes also become an attractive option in cases when a double donation or embryo donor is required, or the desire for secrecy produces an attitude of 'no one has to know'—including, in some cases, the child.

In other cases, people seek gametes in countries where legislation does not regulate certain procedures, such as multiple embryo transfers and sex selection (see Chapter 16, 'ART Regulations and Ethical Guidelines'). For others, the decision simply comes down to the fact that costs are lower in some foreign countries.

While all of these possible benefits might seem a great option, it's important to be aware of the potential risks of undergoing ART treatment in a foreign country—for your and, arguably more importantly, for your child's health.

Conception

Unless you conceive via artificial insemination in a foreign country with your international sperm donor, you will need to undergo some form of ART treatment within your chosen overseas country and/or at your Australian clinic. In the case of conception using egg and embryo donors, you will always be required to undergo ART treatment.

Methods of accessing international donor gametes

There are several ways in which you can access international donor gametes and embryos. You can:

1. access imported frozen gametes via an Australian fertility clinic
2. travel to a foreign country to access gametes and embryos, but use the services of an Australian clinic for the initial part of the treatment
3. travel to foreign countries to independently access both treatment and gametes/embryos.

Let's look at each of these options in more detail.

1 Accessing imported frozen gametes via an Australian fertility clinic

If you decide you want to use an international donor via an Australian clinic, you will need to first check whether your chosen clinic has a service agreement with an international sperm/egg bank (or with multiple banks, in some instances). All processes and procedures that take place (for example, counselling, reimbursements to donor, or family limits) should comply with Australian standards and are audited accordingly (see Chapter 7, 'Choosing an Australian Fertility Clinic').

How does it work?

When obtaining international donor gametes, much of the process is the same as it would be for an Australian clinic-recruited donor, except that the gametes arrive in a cryogenic container and are delivered directly to your chosen clinic's freezer.

You will be required to attend appointments with your fertility specialist and other relevant staff to discuss treatment protocols, attend counselling sessions and a review, be subjected to a cooling-off period (if relevant), select your donor and undergo ART treatment (see Chapter 11, 'Assisted Reproductive Technology [ART], "At-home" Insemination, Success Rates and Costs').

Despite a great deal of similarities to the Australian clinic-recruited donor process, there are a few significant differences, some of which warrant your serious consideration. These are outlined under the following headings.

Counselling

To ensure international donors used by Australian clinics meet our country's standards, Australian clinics are responsible for ensuring that donor counselling has been completed.

Screening

International donors used by Australian clinics should be screened in a manner that meets Australian standards. Checking whether this occurs in an effective manner in all instances may be a worthwhile exercise.

Gamete quality

For more information about gamete quality and ART treatment, see Chapter 11, 'Assisted Reproductive Technology [ART], "At-home" Insemination, Success Rates and Costs'.

ID Release and choosing your donor

Depending on the country in which the sperm/egg bank is located, you might notice when selecting an international donor from a website that not all donors are classified as ID Release. Some may even be listed as 'anonymous'. When importing international gametes to an Australian clinic, you are *only* able to select a donor whose status is ID Release.

The method by which you select your international donor can also vary depending on your clinic. Some options are arguably better than others (see Chapter 7, 'Choosing an Australian Fertility Clinic').

Double donation

If you require a sperm donor and an egg donor, an overseas egg bank *may* also have access to sperm donors. Depending on the policies of both your Australian clinic and the overseas sperm/egg bank(s), the gametes are either fertilised at the international clinic or are shipped to Australia separately to be fertilised at your Australian clinic.

Family limits

When using an international donor, be sure to ask your Australian clinic about family limits. While there are restrictions on family limits in Australia, international sperm/egg banks generally have their own—in many cases, fanciful—*worldwide* family limits. How the two intersect can be a complex and unreliable arrangement (see Chapter 9, 'Choosing Your Donor[s]').

Treatment

Once you have undergone all the requisite steps, your gametes have arrived and the clinic has staff availability, your ART treatment will commence. The type of treatment you undergo will be determined by both you and your fertility specialist (see Chapter 11, 'Assisted Reproductive Technology [ART], "At-home" Insemination, Success Rates and Costs').

2 Travel to a foreign country to access gametes/embryos, with initial treatment in Australia

> *I think anonymous agreements make things 'less messy' for the clinic. It's in their best (financial) interests to keep parties separate and unknowable to each other. It also benefits parents who intend to mislead their children about their true origins. Speaking as the product of 'anonymous' sperm donation, I would encourage you to work with an agency that understands the value of open donations for the donors, parents and children.*
>
> **Erin Jackson (founder of We Are Donor Conceived)**

If you don't wish to import donor gametes to an Australian clinic and are prepared to travel to a foreign country, international egg agencies and sperm banks make this possible in many countries around the world. The process usually involves completing some of your fertility treatment in Australia, then doing a fly-in/fly-out type of arrangement to complete an embryo transfer in a foreign country.

While this may seem like a great option and, no doubt, the agency genuinely has your baby plans as their leading agenda item, it is important to understand that many countries only offer the option of anonymous donors. Sometimes a guarantee of 'total anonymity' is expressed by international clinics in a reassuringly earnest voice promising that the 'biological and emotional issue' of your child having been created with the assistance of another human being's gametes will be thoroughly swept under the proverbial carpet. In many cases, a variety of terms are offered up, such as 'non-identifiable', 'unidentifiable' or 'non-ID release'. Be aware that these all just mean 'anonymous'.

Fundamental to the provision of ART services is that 'patients and their offspring remain the most important consideration in all decisions'.[26] So, while a fertility specialist can assist an intended parent who has made an independent decision to use an international donor, an Australian specialist must not promote or recommend the use of any practices in foreign countries that are considered unethical or illegal in Australia[27] (for example, donor anonymity). To do so would be a breach of the National Health and Medical Research Council (NHMRC) *Ethical Guidelines* (see Chapter 7, 'Choosing an Australian Fertility Clinic'). Arguably more important is the fact that selecting an anonymous donor does not uphold the NHMRC's *Ethical Guidelines* which state that: 'Persons born from donated gametes are entitled to know the details of their genetic origins.'[28]

For more information on anonymity, see Chapter 16, 'ART Regulations and Ethical Guidelines'.

Initial treatment by an Australian clinic

Most people who travel overseas to undergo ART treatment are seeking egg, embryo or double donation. Many of the processes involved are similar to those experienced when dealing with an Australian clinic (see Chapter 4, 'Clinic-recruited Donors').

The requirement to travel overseas introduces elements of planning, logistics and coordination that, for some, might not feel too complicated. But, for others, these can be stressful and overwhelming.

There are many factors to consider, starting with the unknown elements about the donor's fertility. For instance:

- if you are undergoing egg donation, how many eggs will the donor produce and of what quality?
- how many of the eggs will fertilise successfully and how many embryos will be suitable for freezing?
- what if there are no viable embryos?
- if you are undergoing double donation, will the clinic be transparent about the quality of the sperm?
- if you are seeking embryo donation, will the embryos be genetically screened prior to transfer?
- did the people who created the embryos provide consent for their donation?

These factors, combined with the fact that you have flown to another country to undergo ART treatment, can cause significant concern.

How does it work?

> ***Note:*** The following outline is a general guide only. Processes, and the order in which they occur, will vary between countries, clinics and agencies.

Select an Australian fertility specialist

The first step in the process is finding an Australian fertility specialist who is willing to support your attempts at overseas conception because, although the majority of the ART treatment will take place overseas, *prior to* getting on a plane you will be required to prepare for your ART treatment by taking medication and (potentially) undergoing blood tests and ultrasound monitoring scans in Australia. You may also require follow-up support when you arrive home after treatment.

It may be possible to avoid engaging an Australian fertility specialist and to interact solely with your general practitioner (GP). (See 'Treatment protocol' later in this chapter).

However, the possible implications of operating in this way are that you will, in all likelihood, be placed on a 'one-size-fits-all' protocol and may subsequently arrive in your chosen country only to find your treatment can't proceed due to medical reasons (see Chapter 11, 'Assisted Reproductive Technology [ART], "At-home" Insemination, Success Rates and Costs').

Select a country and clinic/agency

The next step is to determine the country (or countries) to which you would be willing to travel (see Chapter 8, 'Choosing an International Sperm/Egg Bank, or Egg Agency'). Once you have identified these, you also need to identify suitable clinics and egg or embryo agencies that exist within those countries. In some instances, you may be required to select the clinic first and the clinic will then direct you to their affiliated agencies for selection of a donor. Some countries have multiple agencies and some may have better processes than others. Alternatively, if the clinic you select has its own pool of donors, you will not be required to use an agency.

Select an international fertility specialist

Whether you are able to select your own fertility specialist in your chosen country depends on the local processes. In some countries, it may be possible for you to select a specialist prior to your departure. In others you might be provided with a handful of options from the relevant clinic upon arrival and asked to make a selection or, in other cases, a specialist will be allocated to you.

Donor selection

Depending on the country you choose, you will either select your own donor or, in countries where all donors are anonymous, the donor may be selected on your behalf (see Chapter 8, 'Choosing an International Sperm/Egg Bank, or Egg Agency'). If you are using your partner's fresh sperm to conceive, both of you will be required to travel to the country you choose.

Confirm donor availability and pay fees

Confirmation of a donor's availability will vary depending on the country you have chosen and the processes required there. For example, in countries where donors are chosen on your behalf, sometimes clinics/agencies have multiple egg donors available but the donors don't always show up for the egg transfer. This means you could receive eggs from whoever is available at the time and also means you might need to stay longer than expected in your chosen country.

In countries in which the process is more structured/regulated and donors are accessed via agencies, the agency will confirm the availability of the egg donor once you have made a selection. You are usually required to pay the donor fee and clinic fee a short time thereafter (often within one week).

Once you have paid the fees, the clinic normally becomes your first point of contact, although the agency might continue to assist you with various aspects of the process and will usually have a timeframe within which you are required to complete your fresh embryo cycle; this is generally three or four months, but might be extended depending on the circumstances.

If you are using frozen embryos, the timeframe may be significantly shorter.

Double donation

If you are undergoing double donation, you will be required to select a sperm donor as well as an egg donor. Depending on the country and the agency, you will either be restricted to local donors from the country in which you are undergoing ART treatment or you may be able to import sperm from other countries around the world.

If you intend to import sperm from another country, you may be required to complete an import permit (see Chapter 8, 'Choosing an International Sperm/Egg Bank, or Egg Agency').

Donor screening

In the case of egg donation, once your donor has agreed and you have paid your fees, the donor is required to attend the clinic to undergo screening (see Chapter 13, 'Being a Donor and How it Works'). If you are using embryo donors, the embryos may undergo genetic screening but this will depend on the accepted processes in the chosen country.

Treatment protocol

Once donor screening has been carried out and the results approved, the foreign clinic will provide you with a treatment plan and corresponding dates (see Chapter 11, 'Assisted Reproductive Technology [ART], "At-home" Insemination, Success Rates and Costs'). The clinic will also usually allocate a specific nurse or staff member with whom you will communicate via ongoing emails, phone conversations or other alternative messaging options.

Prior to your departure from Australia, your Australian fertility specialist will arrange access to the necessary medication and might also recommend an ultrasound, to ensure the endometrium (the lining of your uterus) is thick enough to support conception and pregnancy. If deemed necessary, the dosage of your medication might be altered.

Depending on the country to which you travel, you might also be asked to provide letters from: your GP to confirm basic health indicators, such as blood pressure, have been checked; an obstetrician to ensure you will have appropriate care during pregnancy; and a psychologist to ensure you understand the implications of conceiving a child with a donor.

Counselling

Counselling for donors and intended parents is mandatory in Australia. The same is not true in many other countries. If you are undertaking the first part of your ART treatment in Australia and the remainder in a foreign country, you may miss out on the counselling component. Alternatively, the quality of the counselling could be significantly inferior, or espouse harmful narratives such as, 'Anonymity is best for everyone,' or, 'It's okay *not* to tell your children they are donor-conceived'.

Speak to your fertility specialist about arranging a quality session with an experienced counsellor in Australia before you head overseas.

Payment

The time and manner in which you pay will be determined by the international clinic where you undergo treatment and/or the agency through which you select your donor. International providers usually supply a quote before you leave Australia. If you have selected your donor via an agency, you will be required to pay the agency for the donor and make a separate payment to the clinic for the treatment cycle and embryo creation. This payment to the clinic may or may not include one year's worth of embryo freezing costs.

Any prescription drugs required following your treatment cycle are usually provided in the country where you undergo treatment and are paid for separately. Of course, you will also need to pay your Australian clinic for the part of your treatment cycle that you undergo prior to travelling.

Travel arrangements

Once your treatment plan is locked in, you will need to arrange leave from work (if applicable) and book flights and accommodation in your destination country. In many cases, the international egg agency or clinic will assist you with this process and provide suggestions for local hotels, airport transfers, and so on. You will also need to check whether you require a visa to enter the country. There could also be other considerations, such as your vaccination status.

The term 'locked in' should be used lightly, as things can unravel quickly and create a subsequent need to reschedule. This could not only include changes to your treatment plan but also to your leave from work, your accommodation and your flights so, when making reservations, it is best to consider travel options with flexible payment arrangements.

Some examples of when treatment might need to be rescheduled include yourself or the donor becoming unwell or having to attend an unforeseen event; unsuccessful thickening of the lining of your uterus (see Chapter 11, 'Assisted Reproductive Technology [ART], "At-home" Insemination, Success Rates and Costs'); a change of circumstances at your place of employment meaning your leave cannot be granted; political unrest in your destination country; a pandemic . . .

Appointment at an international fertility clinic

Once you've arrived in your chosen country, you will be required to attend an appointment with a local fertility specialist to check that you are on track for a successful embryo transfer. The egg donor will also have an appointment around the same time to ensure their readiness for egg retrieval.

Embryo transfer

The donor will undergo egg retrieval and, subsequently, all viable eggs will be fertilised with either your donor's prepared sperm or a fresh sperm sample provided by your partner at the clinic. The chosen embryo(s) will be transferred into your uterus and any other viable embryos will be frozen and stored at the clinic.

> ***Note:*** While Australia has strict rules regarding how many embryos can be transferred, some countries do not. This increases the risk of multiple births and premature birth (with the possibility of severe complications for the babies) and other related risks. (See Chapter 16, 'ART Regulations and Ethical Guidelines'). Ensure you do your homework and speak up about your requirements.

Follow up

You may (or may not) be required to stay around for a few days so that the local fertility specialist can monitor the condition of the embryos, called blastocysts at this early stage. You will be provided with medication to support your pregnancy for the short-term.

Additional payments

Depending on the country and the clinic you attend, there may be additional payments required during your treatment process. In some cases, these may not have been previously mentioned. Costs might include post-treatment medication and annual fees for the freezing of any excess embryos. Ensure you check these kinds of details with the clinic upfront, so you do not find yourself in a difficult financial position while overseas.

Back home

Once you are back home, all monitoring can be continued with your Australian fertility specialist.

Further cycles

If you are unsuccessful in achieving a pregnancy or a live birth and you still have frozen embryos created from the treatment cycle, you can use the embryos to undergo a frozen embryo transfer at a later date. However, Australia does not allow for the import of gametes and embryos that do not comply with Australian standards, so you may need to return to the same country to undergo further ART treatment (see Chapter 16, 'ART Regulations and Ethical Guidelines').

While doing your research, you might come across Australian organisations that function in a similar manner to Australian *clinics*, however, such organisations will, for a fee, assist intended parents with many of the challenges of dealing with international providers, such as: communicating and liaising with overseas sperm/egg banks and agencies on your behalf; arranging medication, ultrasounds, blood tests; and so on. By all accounts, a genuine hand-holding exercise. And while it might sound appealing, it's important to be aware that this type of arrangement *may* result in you travelling to a country where all donors are anonymous. Please consider what this means for your donor-conceived child (see Chapter 16, 'ART Regulations and Ethical Guidelines').

For more information on international donors see Chapter 8, 'Choosing an International Sperm/Egg Bank, or Egg Agency'.

3 Independent travel to a foreign country

Sometimes people travel to a foreign country to undergo donor conception without any support at all from an Australian clinic. In other words, the whole end-to-end process of donor conception is conducted at a foreign clinic, including screening. This arrangement might be chosen when a person or their partner has previously lived in another country or has relatives living there and feels comfortable with the local processes. Alternatively, the intended parents may have had a recommendation from someone else who had a successful pregnancy, or they might feel the other country offers them something they cannot obtain in Australia.

How does it work?

Is it safe? Is it worth it? That depends on the country, the standards of medical care, the donor screening process, the ethical standards of the sperm/egg bank or agency, the local legislation regarding ART and donor conception (if any), as well as many other factors—some of which could affect the health of your future child. In all cases, it is recommended you do your homework thoroughly, talk to others who have attended the country and the clinic you are considering, identify the risks and make an informed decision.

For more information on international donors see Chapter 8, 'Choosing an International Sperm/Egg Bank, or Egg Agency'.

6
Known Donors

I found an egg donor on a site where donors meet recipients, and we became good friends. She has four sisters and we're all like sisters; my daughter is their niece. I wanted my daughter to know the donor and have family and relationships—we're family.

Australian recipient parent

What is a known donor?

As the name suggests, a known donor is someone you know, or a person whom you source yourself, *outside* of a clinic. The extent to which you know the person may vary significantly—and, in some cases, the only contact a recipient parent might have with their known donor is via the internet. However, the same principles apply regardless of the situation.

The person might be your partner's sibling, a relative, a friend or an acquaintance, or may be someone you find via a donor matching site (see 'Matching sites' later in this chapter). 'Known donors' can also be referred to as 'private donors', 'recipient-recruited donors', 'patient-recruited donors', 'directed donors' or 'personal donors'.

Unlike a clinic-recruited sperm, egg or embryo donor, a known donor can choose whether they want to donate to you. If they wish, they can communicate with you and make a personal decision about whether they believe you will make a good parent and whether your partner or spouse is committed to being the non-biological parent of a donor-conceived child. They can also be selective about the status and type of your relationship, as well as your sexual orientation, religion, politics, or anything else.

Why people use known donors

There are many reasons why people might choose a known donor rather than a clinic-recruited or international donor. These reasons include:

- limited (or no) availability of clinic-recruited donors, meaning long waiting periods
- limited details being available about donors
- the desire to have an ongoing connection with the donor and enable their child to form a relationship with their biological parent(s) from an early age
- the desire to co-parent (see 'Contact versus co-parenting' later in this chapter).

When it comes to sperm donors specifically, some of the reasons people select a known donor are:

- to avoid the prohibitive costs of undergoing ART treatment at a clinic (especially for people whose fertility may be an unknown—something which applies to many LGBTQIA+ and single people)
- to avoid taking fertility medication
- to have the option of using fresh sperm, rather than frozen sperm
- the desire to meet the potential donor in person (rather than view their details on a computer or in a booklet), get to know them and then make a very intuitive and personal decision about whether the donor is right for them.

Using a known donor requires some big discussions *before* you engage in conception attempts. These discussions should centre on values, ethics, personal preferences, legal ramifications and medical history—as well as the repercussions for yourselves (you and the known donor), your families and any children that may result from the union.

How does it work?

> *When my son was very young, we met up with the sperm donor. It was incredible—they squatted next to each other and looked identical; my son even eats the same spicy foods as him. Soon after, I offered my leftover embryos to a friend*

and she now has two children. So we all catch up regularly; the donor, my friend and our kids. It's really beautiful.

Australian recipient parent

Using a known donor has become fairly commonplace in Australia and overseas. In particular, the LGBTQIA+ community have been creating known-donor families for decades, with friends and recommended acquaintances as donors. Many donor-conceived people advocate for known donors because it means children can potentially know and interact with their biological parents from the outset. Of course, not everyone has access to a willing person whom they feel is responsible or sensible enough to provide gametes and create a child. Known donation is not for everyone and it doesn't come without risk.

The type of known donor you require and the method by which you access that person will largely determine your experience. For instance, if you don't know any responsible adults who fit your criteria, using a matching site may be your only alternative—and that may, or may not, be a positive experience (see 'Matching sites' following).

If you require an egg donor, embryo donor, or double donation, there will be elements of the process you can dictate yourself, but then you will also be required to undergo some form of ART treatment at a clinic and will need to subject yourself to the clinic's protocol. The clinic process will be similar to using a clinic-recruited donor (see Chapter 4, 'Clinic-recruited Donors').

If you require a sperm donor, (most of) the rules are yours to make—unless you are required, or elect, to undergo ART treatment at a clinic.

Matching sites

Warning: The internet may contain traces of nuts.

Author uncertain[29]

Before we look at some of the important aspects to consider when using a known donor, let's delve into the world of internet matching sites. Matching sites exist in various forms online and in social media, making it ridiculously simple to find a willing, responsible and mature sperm donor (although whether they are all responsible and mature adults is debatable) and not too difficult, in many cases, to find an egg or embryo donor.

These forums provide a platform for people seeking donors, as well as people who wish to *be* donors. Then, literally, the twain shall meet.

While some may baulk at the idea of trawling through an unregulated website and swiping right on a smartphone app (or other) with the primary objective of selecting a biological parent for their child, others may feel more relaxed about the exercise and, for some, it may feel like the only option available. Many people have made matching sites work very well for them—however, it's important to know that the risk factors for all parties involved increase exponentially.

When using a donor who is sourced from a matching site, there are several additional factors to consider. Many of these are discussed on the following pages.

> **Note:** The following descriptions regarding matching sites provide a general overview only.

Different aspects of matching sites

> *The amount of misogyny, trickery and smut on* [matching] *apps is staggering and they've been especially toxic to me as a survivor of sexual assault. Pressure to use 'natural insemination' is rampant; others will also do PI, or partial insemination, where the donor masturbates and inserts the penis before climax. 'Stuart, 24', really wants to 'naturally impregnate a girl who wants a baby because I have a breeding kink.' 'Adrian, 38', has really good genes but will only do NI* [natural insemination, or sexual intercourse] *for free; AI* [artificial insemination] *costs. 'Russell, 38', is 'unvaccinated not currently donating to anyone vaccinated.' Ugh. He says my Pfizer may change his DNA . . . sexually. Whatever that means. 'Cameron' is a 'super donor' and tells me that women like him too much and there is no donor*

> *but him who would be satisfactory. 'Cameron' seems to be a narcissist. 'Cameron' tells me I need a 'good hard fuck'. The amount of mansplaining, pressure, kink, and fake news on the app is appalling.*
>
> **American donor-conceived adult and recipient parent**

Matching sites vary *enormously* in their professional appearance and feel, their processes and procedures and the manner in which they are moderated. In most cases, despite Australian clinics crying poor about their donor pools, the sites are literally teeming with donors.

Some sites present as 'egg donor' or 'sperm donor' matching sites only—although they may actually provide the option of seeking the alternate gamete provider in a quiet corner of the site. This is usually to assist intended parents who require a double donation and to cater for people who have had unnerving experiences on sperm-donor-only sites.

Some matching sites also double as a support group once people are pregnant or have had their children.

More versatile matching sites might cover all gamete scenarios and enable every conceivable parenting situation: from single gay males wanting to co-parent; trans couples looking for a sperm donor; heterosexual couples looking for embryo donors; and so on.

Depending on the professionalism of the site, moderators are usually quick to respond if something inadmissible is posted. Some sperm donor matching sites even require people to provide identification, largely due to the presence of sexual predators who may have previously been evicted from the site but then attempt to re-join under a different username.

If you've already taken a look at some matching sites, you'll probably agree that Rene Almeling's assessment of the fertility industry's stereotypical approach to gender (see pages 18 and 213) extends itself to matching sites.

First, you might notice there's a slightly different energy on sperm donor matching sites than there is on egg donor sites. For instance, women and people requiring a sperm donor tend to receive multiple offers instantaneously after posting just one scant introduction (especially if they are attractive). They are usually able to make direct approaches to any donors currently listed as available on the site. Occasionally conversations can become aggressive and accusations, or claims relating to an individual's superior knowledge or sperm count, are thrown around but, if the site is run responsibly, moderators intervene quickly. Sometimes people are evicted.

On the other hand, egg donor-matching sites tend to have a softer energy and, in some cases, have slightly different rules. For instance, intended parents are actively encouraged to share a more thorough account of their personal lives and converse with other site members for a much longer period of time before decisions are made. They are also (usually) required to wait until a donor makes them an offer. This is to avoid egg donors being overwhelmed by requests and subsequently changing their minds about donating.

Why is there a difference between sperm and egg donor-matching sites? Sexual predation aside, it comes down to the fact that the reproductive systems of women and people who produce eggs are different from those of people who produce sperm. Being an egg donor requires a significantly higher level of commitment than ejaculating fifty million sperm into a collection cup, fewer children can result from the egg donations and there is an incomparably greater health risk. As a result, the whole process tends to be taken more seriously. Because, well, from multiple perspectives, it is.

On rare occasions, matching sites attract duplicitous donors who see an opportunity to seek financial compensation for their 'donation'; alternatively, out of desperation, sometimes intended parents make offers.

> ***Note:*** It is a serious criminal offence in Australia to buy or sell gametes and embryos and may result in imprisonment (see Chapter 16, 'ART Regulations and Ethical Guidelines').

On the other hand, it's also good to know that both egg and sperm donor-matching sites are literally overflowing with responsible, kind-hearted people who may be willing to donate their precious gametes to you. Nevertheless, depending on your situation, know that you may be required to strap yourself in for the long game and, particularly if you're seeking a sperm donor, get ready for the possibility of a bit of ducking and weaving to achieve your end goal.

Common features of matching sites

Most matching sites have common features, which may include:

- a list of site rules and how they are policed. This aspect can vary significantly between sites and has the potential to impact your physical safety and mental health.
- disclaimers about the risks involved, the importance of educating yourself and of seeking legal advice
- codes of behaviour
- a supportive online community
- resources related to conception, an outline of ART processes, details about insemination kits, ovulation and pregnancy tests, genetic screening and other relevant topics
- recommendations and instructions regarding donor screening.

Facebook and open internet platforms

Some matching sites take place on open online platforms such as Facebook and, while some of these groups may be strictly moderated and claim high success rates, it's important to be aware of both the risks and the benefits.

Risks

Although the online groups are private, unless you set up a bogus profile, your identity (including personal details, photos, comments and your desire to use a donor) is at risk of public exposure. Furthermore, on platforms such as Facebook, you are also able to view the identity of every single member on the site, as well as any existing members who have a connection with your own Facebook friends.

If you feel the need to protect yourself by setting up a bogus profile it may be appropriate to alert the site administrators, so they know you're not a voyeur with ulterior motives.

Benefits

On the other hand, could using a site on a platform such as Facebook actually foster harmonious relationships between its members?

For instance, because members cannot hide behind dubious usernames like 'Sir Cumalot' or 'Master Bator', and everyone can view each other's profiles, in many cases members can take a look at what people are posting on their personal pages and decide whether they like what they see—or not. Members can potentially offer a greater level of genuine support and can observe, call out and report inappropriate behaviour quickly, as well as readily discuss topics of interest, such as insemination kits or ovulation tracking. In some cases, members who live near each other might organise social gatherings for donors and recipient parents to all meet face-to-face.

People advertising for a donor can also ask existing members to respect their privacy if they happen to know who they are. Whether that request will be respected or not is, of course, an unknown and using a platform such as Facebook to find a donor may or may not be for you.

Setting up an account

Users of online platforms generally set up an account and a username that includes:

- an 'intended parent' advertisement (see 'Advertising for a donor' following)
- a profile photo (optional)
- their location
- their status (for example, donor, intended parent, or partner)
- how they wish to receive the donation (for example, AI or ART treatment at a clinic)
- their cycle timing and availability
- parenting and communication requirements (for example, limited or frequent contact, or co-parenting).

Advertising for a donor

If using an online matching site, you will need to place an advertisement outlining what you are seeking. Many matching sites will provide you with tips and suggestions that assist you to create the advertisement. In some cases, you can even submit your draft to the site administrator who will provide you with feedback and further suggestions before you post the final advertisement on the site. To get some ideas, you might also wish to read existing advertisements posted by others.

Sites often suggest that your success in connecting with a donor may depend on the level of detail you provide about yourself. Such details might include:

- a description of yourself (and your partner, if applicable)
- your age
- any other children you have
- your relationship status
- a photo (if you're comfortable providing one)
- the reasons why you are seeking a donor
- whether you're willing to travel for the purposes of the conception process
- the level of contact the donor will be able to have with your future child.

For more information about donor and sibling linking and legislation see Chapter 15, 'Donor and Sibling Linking', and Chapter 16, 'ART Regulations and Ethical Guidelines'.

> ***Note:*** Some states might require you to have your advertisement approved by the Minister for Health before you publish it. Approval can take anywhere up to eight weeks. Make sure you write your advertisement correctly the first time and send the final version to the relevant State (not Federal) Minister for Health.

It's a match!

> *The idea of using a known donor is to have someone who will remain in your life in some capacity, so don't choose anyone who plans to literally just drop sperm off on your doorstep and walk away.*
>
> **Australian donor-conceived adult (NSW)**

What happens when a match occurs?

When a donor makes an offer or accepts a request, or when a donor and a recipient 'like' each other's posts (depending on the site), the parties involved usually take themselves offline and arrange to chat more and, perhaps, meet in person. Communication continues until an agreement is reached, or a decision is made to discontinue. When the latter occurs, the intended parents (and the donor) need to start again.

In some instances, particularly on sites where people have non-identifying profiles, the first time the intended parent and the donor meet is to hand over the sperm sample.

In some cases, the intended parents and donor don't meet at all and the donor simply deposits the sample in a hotel room and then leaves the premises. While this may seem like a simple solution to your baby problems, it's important to remember that this stranger is going to be the biological parent of your child (of course, this doesn't mean they will *parent* your child, in the verb sense). For instance, do you even know whether their profile photos belong to them or whether they're just images sourced from the internet? Is the person you've been chatting with online really a plumber who loves golf and attending women's rights protests, or are they into populating the planet and racial purity, and a lifetime member of the Lads Society?

Probably best to meet up with them, make a personal assessment and do your best to find out, right? Why? Because, whether you like it or not, you (and especially your children and your children's children) are going to be connected to this person forever.

Issues to consider

Following are some questions to help you identify whether using a matching site is for you.

Credibility of the site

- Who set up the site? Is the site owner a donor or recipient wishing to assist others, or are they looking to run a professional income-producing business? It's up to you to decide whether the latter sits comfortably with you.
- To what extent are your personal details protected?
- Can you communicate with other members via personal messages in which details can be exchanged privately?
- Do moderators monitor the site by issuing warnings to offenders and removing inappropriate posts and, on occasion, offenders?
- Are you able to delete your account, or easily remove yourself and your profile from the group at any time?

Trusting your donor

> *I found a donor on a matching site who used a fake name and address. After months of searching, I discovered he's an academic and has conceived about 50 kids. I found all his ads—he has multiple accounts on different sites and uses disgusting names to advertise himself (he didn't when I chose him). I've found many of the families and all the children look the same. I'll never speak negatively about him in front of my daughter, but I just want him to stop. He says I'm the last, but who can really trust the man?*
>
> **Australian recipient parent**

How much do you trust your potential donor? This is something only you can gauge and it is vital you discuss all of your needs with your donor, complete your research and use your intuition to determine whether they are the right person to become the biological parent of your child. An Australian known sperm donor explains, 'It's all done on a handshake agreement. EVERYTHING is about trust—if you don't have trust, you're asking for trouble':

> *If I was going to offer advice to women considering a known donor, I'd say, meet up with them at least once, and in a public place. Then at your first meeting, see if he's brought his recent STI* [sexually transmitted infection] *check,* [and] *his sperm analysis. This would tell me if he's genuine or not. Discuss your expectations and make sure they're the same. By then I would've already checked out his social media pages to see what things he's into and, if there's any weird or aggressive stuff, I'd avoid him at all costs. And if he says he's only into NI* [natural insemination, or sexual intercourse] *or that NI is more effective, I'd run a mile. You've really got to trust your gut.*

Consider the following questions.

- How many existing children does the donor have? How many do they intend to have (including their own)?
- Are there other people on the matching site who have had experience with this donor and can share their opinions with you?
- Does the donor advertise on multiple matching sites?
- Have they previously been (or are they currently) a clinic-recruited donor?
- Has the donor asked for money (other than reimbursement of reasonable out-of-pocket expenses), or do you get the sense you are being groomed to hand over vast amounts of cash at the eleventh hour?
- Is the donor using images of their existing donor-conceived children to advertise themselves, possibly without the relevant recipient parents permission?

Sperm donors

> *If you're not in a hurry, are happy to wait a couple of menstrual cycles and insist on AI* [artificial insemination] *only, this tends to weed out a lot of the dodgy people.*
>
> **Australian recipient parent**

Consider the following questions about sperm donors:

- Have you met your donor in person?
- Do you know the donor's real name? Have you seen some proof of identification, such as their Medicare card (if they have a partner and children, they may also be listed on the Medicare card)?
- Do they wear a wedding ring but refuse to discuss their spouse?
- Do they refuse to undergo a sexually transmitted infection screening check?
- Do they insist on natural insemination (sexual intercourse) when you've indicated you will not consider this under any circumstances?
- Do they insist on natural insemination but have actually had a vasectomy (ask to view their semen analysis)?
- Are they telling you, 'I can get you pregnant, even when you're not ovulating'?
- Do their written responses to you sound generic, as though they've just replied to several people at once?
- Do you have their contact details so you can contact them in the future?

International donors sourced via matching sites

> *I've seen women on some* [international matching] *sites say things like, 'Need a sperm donor next Tuesday. Anyone available?' I mean, I've seen people put more effort into finding a good hairdresser than some of these people put into finding a donor. It's insane. And there's usually plenty of responders. Truly, who even* are *these men?*
>
> **Australian recipient parent**

International matching sites exist in abundance and, if you search hard enough, you'll uncover sites that offer egg donors from India and sperm donors from Brazil; sites that represent specific racial and ethnic groups; donors with PhDs; exceptionally tall donors; and more. While it may seem a tantalising prospect, it's important to know that the risks escalate substantially if you use international matching sites.

Sperm donors

Consider the following questions when making your decision.

- In your donor's country of origin what, if any, are the laws related to known donors? For instance, the use of donor sperm is not permitted in some countries. In others, if a medical professional is not present during the conception process, or if you are single, the donor may be considered to be the legal parent.
- Is your donor providing you with their correct personal details, including their real name? Many known donors on international sites openly admit to using false names—and encourage others to do the same—so they can remain anonymous should their offspring wish to connect them later.
- If your donor resides in another country with different parenting laws, or no relevant laws at all, are you able to arrange and sign a preconception agreement with them? If it can be arranged, will it have any merit?
- Is there a possibility your donor may seek to claim parenting rights to your child?

> ***Note:*** If you intend to import your international donor's sperm from another country to a residential address, it is unlikely to make it through the airport gate. Sperm will not survive for extended periods in a cryogenic container and, if it does, how do you actually know whose swimmers are inside the container?

Egg donors

Due to the complex and invasive procedures involved in egg donation, intended parents who find a known donor on an international matching site will still need to seek ART treatment, either in Australia or in the donor's country of residence. (For more information see Chapter 11, 'Assisted Reproductive Technology [ART], "At-home" Insemination, Success Rates and Costs'.)

Serial sperm donors

> *If you're using a known donor you've met off the internet—do your research. Join Facebook groups and Google them to make sure they are who they say they are. And never use a super donor. They obviously can't have any kind of meaningful relationship with their donor-conceived offspring, and it's not ethical, no matter how badly you want a baby.*
>
> **Australian donor-conceived adult (NSW)**

While the term, 'super sperm donor' or 'serial donor', may offer great promise to an intended parent—suggesting high quality-sperm, excellent success rates and the concept of a large family network—the outcome may not be so attractive for the child you create. If you are feeling frustrated with your clinic, can't afford ART treatment and are feeling inspired to use the latest and greatest serial donor, there are several things of which you need to be aware.

Firstly, what is a serial donor?

Serial donors, sometimes known as 'megadonors' or 'super sperm donors', are self-proclaimed men who embark on elaborate campaigns to create as many children as possible. Different serial donors will have different modus operandi. For instance, a serial donor may hide behind multiple pseudonyms, advertising on several sites to trick intended parents into believing just a handful of children exist. Alternatively, they may be quite blatant about the fact they're aiming for '800 kids by Christmas'. Serial donors might have their own social media profiles where they report their weekly birth tally and current 'tour' locations:

'Two sets of twins born this week and five lucky mamas pregnant!'; or 'Successful week this week with three girls and two boys!' Sometimes serial donors band together in private groups to discuss and compare each other's running totals. Friendly (and, sometimes, not-so-friendly) competition abounds.

Serial donors may offer artificial insemination only (see Chapter 11, 'Assisted Reproductive Technology [ART], "At-home" Insemination, Success Rates and Costs'), or they might encourage natural insemination (sexual intercourse). Some may neglect to mention their wives—people who may not even know about their husband's donation activities and resulting children. Others drive around the country in a van, masturbate in the back and hand over their samples to hopefuls who wait outside.[30] Some start off as clinic-recruited donors and then take up known donation—occasionally on a scale of colossal proportions.[31] Some stay local, while others fly around the globe and strive to deposit their genes in as many countries as possible.[32]

Sometimes serial donors are happy to connect with their children and sometimes they're not; occasionally they're selective. Some parents who conceived via natural insemination have successfully taken their serial donor to court to receive child support—this doesn't necessarily stop the serial donor on their campaign to flood the gene pool.[33]

And obviously, many, many people use them.

The risks of using a serial donor

> *I think there is something unnatural about any one donor having dozens or hundreds of offspring—it's just not how the human gene pool is supposed to work. I can't imagine what the offspring of these internet super donors will think when they eventually begin to wonder about that part of themselves.*
>
> **American donor-conceived adult**

While it may feel simple and convenient to use a fertile serial donor and then walk away to experience your wondrous new life as a parent—feeling thrilled at the notion of such a large family community, or feeling safe that your donor will be far too busy to want any ongoing involvement with you or your child—the problem now lies with your child. Many donor-conceived people express curiosity about the motivation behind the donation—knowing it was done to 'pass on exceptional genes', or to 'maximise genetic diversity' (an erroneous claim) may feel abhorrent. Furthermore, how might they feel about sharing 50% of their DNA with a person who used public recruitment statements like, 'If you've got a spare uterus, I'll do my best to put a baby in there!'? How will they make sense of dozens, or even hundreds, of siblings, many of whom they will never find, let alone meet; or make sense of communicating with the donor whom they may regard as untrustworthy? (For more information on the risks of high sibling numbers, see Chapter 9, 'Choosing Your Donor[s]')

How the risks associated with using a serial sperm donor can be minimised

Unless your known donor is a close friend or relative, the risk of falling for the charms of a serial sperm donor still exists. Furthermore, even if a donor does not originally set out with plans to populate the planet, according to some serial donors making babies is addictive, especially when they start to receive requests from potential recipients on a regular basis. Sadly, there's not much that can be done to stop them, because current legislation does not regulate known donors. Nevertheless, there are several things you can do that *may* minimise the risks of using a serial donor, as listed below.

- Use the internet to educate yourself regarding the names of existing serial donors (some social media groups provide a list of donors who have large numbers of children).
- To check whether the potential donor's name is real or bogus, research the name online by asking questions of people in relevant social media groups.
- Avoid donors who have their own public website or social media page.
- Avoid donors whose social media username includes the word 'donor'. For example, '[insert first name] Donor'.
- Avoid 'dump-and-run' style inseminations, where you don't even get to meet the donor in person.

- Meet with your potential donor on multiple occasions and ask to see identification such as a driver's licence or passport. Get to know the donor and discuss how the arrangement will work (see 'Asking the right questions of your potential donor' following).
- Choose a trustworthy person who is already known to you.

Of course, you may still be happy to go ahead with a serial donor—although it's important to consider whether your child will thank you for it, or not.

Asking the right questions of your potential donor

When communicating with potential donors on matching sites, make sure you are polite and treat them with respect (after all, one of them may become your child's biological parent). Some known donors have described intended parents' initial requests as rude and entitled, making brash introductory statements like: 'Are you available? I want to use your sperm.'

If the donor decides that you won't be a good match, thank them for their time and respectfully move on. Some donors have reported episodes of verbal abuse when they have declined a request.

If you don't want to use a clinic-recruited donor or a social media matching site, and you don't have people offering their gametes to you right now, how do you go about asking someone that you know to be your donor? The answer to this question will depend on how well you know the person and the nature of your relationship with them. For example, have you known them for thirty years, or for thirty minutes? Are they already in a relationship and, if so, do you know their partner? Do they have children of their own? Do they *want* children of their own?

If you are using a known egg donor on a matching site, you will have already had multiple online conversations with your potential donor and, in many cases, site rules stipulate you must wait for the donor to make you an offer.

If you don't wish to ask people directly because you are concerned about the impact it will have on your friendship, you may wish to put the word out to your friends and family that you are considering gamete donation and wait to see who offers. For example, the offer might come from an acquaintance, or from a friend of a friend. Sometimes people have already considered being a donor but have never taken the next step.

In the case of egg donation, some people may be unaware of the intrusive nature of the procedures involved so, if someone expresses willingness to donate eggs, ensure you have a conversation about what is required.[34]

If you decide to ask a friend or acquaintance directly, the following suggestions might help you start the conversation.

- Find a space where you have privacy.
- Have the conversation face-to-face, if possible.
- Be clear that you are serious and that it's not some kind of passing fancy.
- Give them plenty of time to think about it. This *might* be the first time they've even thought about children.
- Give them time to talk about it with their partner (if this applies).
- Be clear about the role, if any, you would want them to play.
- If the conversation doesn't go as planned or things become uncomfortable, let the person go and start the conversation again with someone else.
- Whatever the outcome of the conversation, be sure to thank the person for their time and consideration.

The important thing is not to rush. It could take months for you and a prospective donor to reach a decision and make arrangements regarding the method you'll use, health screening, ongoing contact, and so on.

Don't be offended if your potential donor says 'No'. While many people jump at the chance of being a donor, conceiving a child should be a deliberate, conscious choice by all parties involved and withdrawing from the process is probably better than the donor proceeding with doubts or through a sense of obligation.[35]

Becoming a donor is not for everyone.

Counselling

Sperm donors

When a person elects to use a clinic-recruited or international sperm donor, all parties are required to undergo counselling (unless you are undergoing fertility treatment overseas)—and there is a very good reason for this. First, while many donors are responsible, mature adults, there are also vast numbers who don't fully understand the long-term repercussions of their donations. This is especially true of people who are seeking to saturate the gene pool in their chosen locations.

Understanding the unique needs of donor-conceived children is something frequently missing by those seeking to become recipient parents, yet it is paramount to ensuring the long-term mental and emotional health of a donor-conceived child. When using a known donor, it is important to consider that you and your donor—and all partners—undergo at least one session of counselling with a qualified person.

Egg and embryo donors

If you are using a known egg or embryo donor, you will be required to undergo counselling as part of the Australian clinic's treatment protocol (see Chapter 4, 'Clinic-recruited Donors').

Contact versus co-parenting

> *My advice to anyone who is considering growing their family in this way* [known donation] *would be to really focus on building trust and communication, and to discuss expectations and plan ways to resolve potential conflicts or differences of opinion. There are many people who are making this sort of arrangement work without drama, just as there are people who don't end up in court when their relationships break down.*
>
> **Australian donor-conceived adult (NSW)**

Another essential topic for discussion with your known donor is the level of contact your child might have with them and their partner and family; it's also important to acknowledge that the level of contact may change over time. It is imperative that you and your donor make your intentions clear and agree on conditions *before* beginning attempts to conceive.

At one end of the parenting spectrum there are people who wish to co-parent with their donor; at the other end there are those who want no contact at all; and then there is everything in between. Ensure both (or all) parents, especially the non-biological parent(s), participate in discussions and agree on all terms and conditions.

Co-parenting

What is co-parenting and how does it work?

A person can only co-parent if the law confers parental responsibility. In other words, it's about legal rights and legal obligations. The general rule is that, if a person wants parental rights (time spent with the child), that person also has responsibilities (for example, making decisions about things like immunisations, religion, schools, etc.). These rights and responsibilities are conferred on both parents. Conversely, choosing to have no rights equals no responsibilities.

The law generally contemplates co-parenting in post-relationship terms, that is, when two people have separated. This is obviously different from a donor conception scenario. Recipient parents and donors who wish to co-parent should seek legal advice to outline the nature of their co-parenting arrangements and the shared parental responsibility. If things become 'messy' in the relationship, the 'best interests of the child' will be the determining factor in a court.

In all situations, ensure you seek legal advice about the roles each adult will play in your child's life and outline the nature of the arrangements in a preconception agreement *before* conception attempts begin—again, noting that this may change over time (see Chapter 16, 'ART Regulations and Ethical Guidelines').

Possible topics for discussion with your known donor about co-parenting

- Will your donor be involved during pregnancy and birth—and to what extent?
- Will your donor have any input in naming your child?
- How much time will your child spend at the donor's (and their partner's) house, and how much time at yours? Will you go on holidays together?
- What style of parenting do you prefer in early infancy? For instance, do you prefer attachment parenting and co-sleeping, while your donor believes in three-hourly bottle feeds and a cot in the upstairs bedroom?
- What about education and schooling? Does your donor prefer the local private school where every child has a laptop in Grade 1, while you want to home-school?
- Do you want your child to be television-free, while your donor is keen to live stream *Peppa Pig* directly from iPad to pram?
- If you are single now, will you feel the same way about co-parenting with your known donor if you find a partner in the future?
- If you separate from your partner, how will you manage the relationship breakdown in terms of your child's needs?
- If your donor has a partner, what role will that person, and their extended family, play in the co-parenting arrangement for your child?
- If your donor re-partners at some stage, how will you feel about their new partner having contact with your child?

General contact

> *My known donor has worked out so well! There are four babies and three of us get together every two months. We see the donor about once a month to say hi, and we exchange small presents. I also send postcards to his mum who lives overseas. Using a known donor has 100% been the right decision for me.*
>
> **Australian recipient parent**

If you do not intend to co-parent, what does contact with your child's biological parent look like for you?

Some donor-conceived people feel strongly that the only way to ethically participate in donor conception involves the use of a donor who has ongoing contact with their child. This is usually to minimise issues regarding genetic mirroring and identity development; minimise the potential grief of not knowing a biological parent; and to facilitate easy access to familial medical history (see Chapter 9, 'Choosing Your Donor[s]'). For some people this is an alarming concept and very different from the industry narrative which, on occasion, asserts that 'the donor is just providing a cell'.

So, how do you balance the needs of your child and the needs of your donor?

Having a connection with your donor does not necessarily mean they will play an active role in parenting your child. Contact might just involve catch-ups, attendance at celebrations and special events such as birthdays or sporting events, and even getting to know members of extended family such as cousins and grandparents.

The important thing is to ensure that you and your donor agree. If you are very clear from the outset about what you want and it does not match your known donor's requirements, it would probably be a good idea to find another donor. Alternatively, if you make an agreement to include your donor in your child's life and then change your mind at the eleventh hour, be aware that this can have potentially devastating effects for all parties involved.

Possible topics for discussion with your known donor about contact

Following are some points that might assist you to establish the amount and type of contact between the donor and the child.

- What level of contact will your known donor have after your child is born and as they grow older?
- Will contact commence early in the child's life, or will you introduce contact gradually and see how it goes?
- Will the contact be sporadic or regular; once a week; once a year?

- Will the known donor be transparent about the role they played in your child's birth and discuss it openly with their own partner, family, children and friends? What will any relationships with these people look like?
- Will you share photos and celebrate special events, such as birthdays, social or cultural events, religious holidays, and so on?
- If your known donor has their own children (or intends to have children later), how will they feel about their parent being a donor? Do they even know?
- How will your child refer to the donor and their partner? (For more information about language and terminology see Chapter 14, 'Talking about Donor Conception'.)

Other considerations are discussed under the headings which follow.

Preconception agreement

Regardless of your situation, it's important to be aware that, if your known donor spends time with your donor-conceived child and a dispute arises, parental rights are likely to be recognised if the court decides that continued contact is in the best interests of the child. Obtaining a preconception agreement and seeking legal advice before going ahead with a known donor is a very good idea. (For more information about preconception agreements and parenting orders see Chapter 16, 'ART Regulations and Ethical Guidelines'.)

Lifestyle preferences

For more information about how your lifestyle preferences and those of your donor need to be a consideration see Chapter 9, 'Choosing Your Donor[s]'.

Finances: Who pays?

For more information about the financial obligations of the parties to donor conception see Chapter 9, 'Choosing Your Donor[s]'.

Family limits and siblings

For more information about family limits and numbers of siblings see Chapter 9, 'Choosing Your Donor[s]'.

Conception

Sperm donors

If you choose a known sperm donor, you would be advised to attend a health screening centre to undergo all the requisite testing, as well as ART procedures such as artificial insemination. Some intended parents may know from the outset that they will be required to undergo ART treatment. The treatment might be as simple as medication to stimulate ovulation, or as extensive as a full IVF cycle (see Chapter 11, 'Assisted Reproductive Technology [ART], "At-home" Insemination, Success Rates and Costs').

Fertility clinics are required to collect and maintain records of each known donor, any children born and the intended parent's identifying information. They must pass on this information to the relevant state or territory's donor register, if one exists (see Chapter 15, 'Donor and Sibling Linking'). Your known donor might also be required to sign documentation indicating they do not have an intention to claim parenting rights.

If you are not using a clinic, one of the most important decisions to make is the location of your conception attempts. Depending on the relationship you have with your known donor, you may wish to attempt conception in your own home or at a neutral location, such as a motel. Some people stay overnight at a motel and receive a second (or third) donation the next day. Others make a brief holiday of it.

If you choose to undergo artificial insemination at home (or at another location), the act of conception requires open communication channels between you and your donor, particularly concerning the timing of events. For instance, the donor will need to know when your cycle commences and when you're ready for an attempt at conception (or multiple attempts in the one cycle). They will also need to know whether the attempt(s) were successful or whether you wish to try again.

While there are benefits to conceiving via artificial insemination 'at home', including reduced risk of gamete environmental degeneration and, for some, the fact that their child was conceived at home rather than in a laboratory, there are also many risk factors. Some of these include your physical safety, your mental health, your sexual health, your legal rights and, arguably the most important aspect of all, the health and wellbeing of your child (including inherited medical conditions). Another important factor to consider is whether your known sperm donor is actually producing good-quality sperm, so having their sperm tested beforehand is a good idea.

In all situations, it is imperative you create a foundation of open communication. Establish clear boundaries with your donor around your needs and preferences during the conception process, do not compromise on anything that impacts your mental, emotional and physical wellbeing (for example, aggressive and sexually predatory behaviour) and, if you are a single person, you might consider having a support person with you. If you have a partner (or partners) who will be non-biological parents, they may wish to assist with the insemination process.

Be aware that, if you conceive via natural insemination (sexual intercourse with the donor), there is a much greater risk that the law will consider your sperm donor to be a legal parent of your donor-conceived child (see Chapter 16, 'ART Regulations and Ethical Guidelines'). This is because it is presumed that, if the parties consent to an artificial conception procedure, the intention is to 'opt out' of the legal parental responsibility which the *Family Law Act 1975* (Cth) automatically confers to the parents of a child conceived naturally. As a consequence of this, conceiving via sexual intercourse is strongly recommended against by everyone in 'officialdom'. However, undeterred by this legality, through lack of knowledge, unfailing trust in their donor, unwavering confidence in their sexuality, or for some other reason, people still use this method.

If you find yourself actually considering natural insemination, apart from the aforementioned legal issues, consider the possibility that significant long-term complications could arise after your child is born. For example, will your emotional and mental health (and that of your future child) be impacted should your donor seek to be identified as the legal father of your child in a court?

> *I was very clear on my profile that I only wanted to do the AI* [artificial insemination] *method and only ever chose donors who wanted the same. However, two donors we met up with tried to persuade us on the day that NI* [natural insemination] *would be better and that I was more likely to get pregnant this way. We just left immediately. It was so infuriating and pretty creepy to be honest.*
>
> **Australian recipient parent**

If you originally agreed on artificial insemination, but your donor attempts to convince you on the day that natural insemination is 'the only way', or 'it's just a medical procedure', or 'don't worry, it will be over quickly', consider the option of walking away and choosing a different donor—as well as reporting the donor to the administrator on your matching site and completing a police report if you believe a sexual assault has taken place.

> *You wouldn't believe how convincing some of these guys are, especially when women are desperate to get pregnant. One guy I know of used to promise women that if they did NI* [natural insemination], *they'd get a result first time. He would even convince married women and lesbians to sleep with him.*
>
> **Australian known sperm donor**

While many stories abound on the internet about known donors handing their semen sample over to recipients in Target bathrooms or from the rear door of a white van, it's important to consider how this act of conception might impact your child should they ask for the details later. Some donor-conceived people already feel grief and trauma about their conception story. If your child or teen asks about the facts of their conception, the addition of a public bathroom, a stranger and a specimen cup may not be received well—will you feel comfortable revealing the truth?

Another important thing to consider is that, if you don't trust your donor to visit your home or feel safe during the conception process, are they really the right person to be the biological parent of your child?

Egg and embryo donors

If you require an egg or embryo donor, regardless of the type of donor you select, you will need to undergo some form of ART treatment at a clinic. To facilitate this, you will be guided by your clinic's protocols and your own personal experiences and preferences. For instance, if your egg donor lives a long way away from you, or even interstate, which one of you will travel? If your donor has previously donated, do they have a preference for clinics or specialists or, conversely, a list of clinics and specialists they refuse to work with due to a previous poor experience?

Topics for discussion with your known sperm donor about conception attempts

Some topics for discussion between you and your known donor (and their partner, if applicable) might include some from the following list.

- Is the donor willing to undergo a sperm analysis? If so, are they willing to provide you with a copy of the results so you can make your own assessment of their suitability as a donor?

  Andrology laboratories specialise in sperm analysis and may be a better option than a pathology laboratory.[36]

- At what point prior to the conception attempt will you accept your donor's 'current' health screening tests (make sure they are authentic). These might include a urine test, blood tests and tests for sexually transmitted infections. Obtain a sample of the list of tests completed by clinics if you are unsure.

  A donor may ask to see your relevant test results as well.

- What location is acceptable to both of you for the conception attempt(s)?
- Who will be present when the conception attempt occurs?
- How many conception attempts would you like to undergo for the cycle? Is your donor willing to accommodate your needs if, for

example, you wish to undergo artificial insemination twice or three times during your cycle?

- Is your donor undergoing multiple conception attempts with other people, or just focusing on you? (This might impact the quality of the sperm.)
- If your attempts at conception are unsuccessful, would your donor be open to the possibility of undergoing IVF (see Chapter 11, 'Assisted Reproductive Technology [ART], "At-home" Insemination, Success Rates and Costs')?
- What will you do with any unused embryos should you decide to undergo IVF?

Topics for discussion with your known egg donor about conception attempts

- How does the donor think donation of their eggs might impact their relationship with their own partner?
- Is the donor familiar with the procedures they will need to undergo, including the drug protocol?
- Which clinic will you both attend to undergo ART treatment?
- Are you both comfortable with the specialist who will complete the treatment?

Topics for discussion with your known embryo donor about conception attempts

- Has any genetic screening been conducted on the embryo donor(s) (see Chapter 9, 69Choosing Your Donor[s])?
- What would you like to happen to any excess embryos (see Chapter 9, 'Choosing Your Donor[s]', and Chapter 11, 'Assisted Reproductive Technology [ART], "At-home" Insemination, Success Rates and Costs')?

For more information about the IVF process, see Chapter 11, 'Assisted Reproductive Technology [ART], "At-home" Insemination, Success Rates and Costs'.

Part Three: Making Decisions

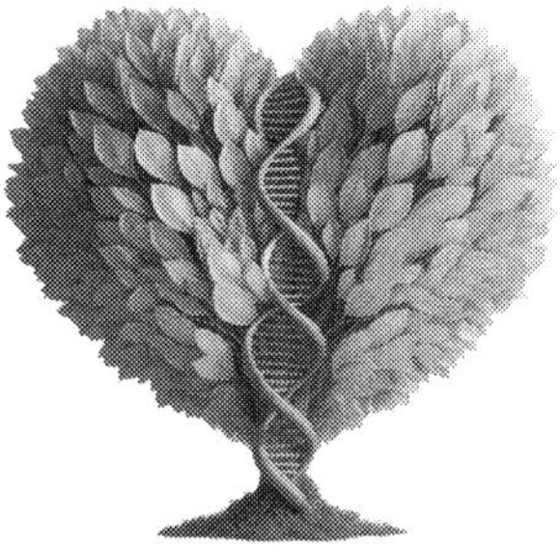

Whatever you plan to do, make sure you can truthfully answer all [of your child's] questions about your choices. Be prepared to have answers as to how you came to your decisions, why you made such choices, how you made agreements—honest answers, not romanticised ones.

Australian recipient parent

The next four chapters outline some of the things you might wish to consider when making your decisions and, more importantly, may help you to identify those factors that are in the best interests of your child. Best of luck with your decisions (none of which should be taken lightly) and know that whatever decisions you make will change your life, and the life of your future child, forever.

If you're not quite ready to make decisions about choosing a clinic, an agency or a donor, skip this part and come back to it later.

7

Choosing an Australian Fertility Clinic

If I were to give advice to potential parents, I'd say research the clinics and doctors and avoid those that have bad reputations and practices, avoid getting caught up in the numbers regarding eggs retrieved, talk to donors about how they've been treated and know that cheaper is not always better.

Ashley Ford (Australian egg donor and moderator of the Egg Donation Australia website)

> ***Note:*** Even if you are not considering using a fertility clinic at this point, reading this chapter is worthwhile to help you understand what clinics offer, in case you require assistance with conception or pregnancy at a later stage, or if you decide to take your known sperm donor to a clinic to undergo screening.

Just as you might refer to *Choice* magazine to decide which vacuum cleaner is the most effective and practical for your new multi-level loop pile carpet, so too can you read *Choice*'s reports on various aspects of Australian fertility clinics, including success rate data and treatment costs.[37]

In 2016, the Australian Competition and Consumer Commission (ACCC) investigated the rather large disparity in the success rates of fertility clinics and found that some of the results being advertised were misleading and used ambiguous and confusing terminology. As a result of the investigation, the ACCC issued a warning to fertility clinics, directing them to tidy up their language and reporting data, ensuring customers are able to make informed decisions about treatment options.[38]

In 2017, it was revealed via an annual report that some clinics offered their specialists a $500,000 bonus if they performed over four hundred IVF cycles each year for three consecutive years, 'acknowledging the value they generate for shareholders'.[39]

In 2019, the Health Complaints Commissioner (HCC) conducted an Inquiry into ART practices in Victoria with the findings indicating that clinics are falling short in multiple areas, including communication, advertising, counselling and complaint handling. Subsequent recommendations have been made.[40]

I'm sure you're getting the picture . . .

Without a doubt, there are hardworking, genuine, principled individuals within the industry who will always have your best interests at heart. Perhaps this individual is your fertility specialist, your embryologist, your donor coordinator, your nurse. Perhaps *all* of the people in your team are ethical and responsible. But what about others with vested interests—the ones discussing corporate policy; annual profits; shareholder equity; and capital growth? Will they be concerned about your cancelled ART cycle because the donor's sperm count turned out to be significantly lower than claimed? Or the fact that your fertility specialist won't answer your calls . . . or the matter of your child being created with the wrong donor's sperm?

Australian clinics have beautifully presented, user-friendly websites covering what's involved in starting a family, glossy images of lab technicians and newborn babies, available fertility options and associated costs. There are slick looking brochures available on request; metaphorically symbolic logos; fact sheets; data related to how many babies the clinic has produced; statements about cutting edge science and technology, LGBTQIA+ advocacy; and free information sessions you can attend.

Shiny objects aside, and irrespective of the method you use to select your donor, if you attend a clinic for any part of the conception process there are several things you need to consider. Some of these will be discussed on the following pages.

Accreditation of ART and national guidelines

Arguably, the most important thing to check when using a fertility clinic or independent fertility specialist is whether they are accredited (this will usually be highlighted on their website somewhere). This single fact alone may—with absolutely no guarantees—prevent you from experiencing potentially disastrous outcomes such as losing all of your embryos if the power to your clinic's storage container fails,[41] or discovering too late that the abnormal embryos you chose to destroy were actually normal.[42]

How does it all work?

The Fertility Society of Australia and New Zealand (FSANZ)

The Fertility Society of Australia and New Zealand (FSANZ) is the peak body for reproductive medicine in Australia and New Zealand, representing scientists, doctors, researchers, nurses, counsellors and consumers.

The FSANZ is responsible for setting the standards for the practice of fertility medicine across Australia. Some of the society's objectives include: improving the standard of reproductive medical practices and fertility services offered; encouraging research into reproductive health; providing educational opportunities for FSANZ members to raise the standard of care.[43]

The Reproductive Technology Accreditation Committee (RTAC)

The Reproductive Technology Accreditation Committee (RTAC) is a subcommittee of the Board of FSANZ, made up of expert representatives from all specialty areas of ART, including reproductive medicine, nursing, counselling and reproductive biology. This committee reports directly to the FSANZ Board and also includes representation from NZ fertility consumer organisations. Australian clinics carrying out ART treatments are required to be accredited by the RTAC and it is the RTAC that sets the standards for:

- the performance of ART
- accreditation and auditing of ART centres

- promotion of continuous improvement to the quality of care received by people undergoing ART treatment.

The RTAC *Code of Practice*

The *Code of Practice for Assisted Technology Units* is a document developed by the RTAC to set and maintain minimum standards for clinics or centres offering ART, and to ensure ART clinics comply with the ART laws and guidelines.

What it means to be 'RTAC certified'

Assisted reproductive technology is made up of many processes, including clinical treatments, counselling services, and laboratory procedures for the assessment and preparation of human gametes and embryos.[44] Compliance with the RTAC *Code of Practice* is mandatory for organisations involved in the treatment of patients using any or all of these ART procedures.

An initial audit of standards and practices is carried out to determine whether an ART provider meets the standards required to be RTAC certified. All registered providers of ART are then regularly audited to ensure continued compliance with the RTAC *Code of Practice* and to check they fulfil the specific criteria necessary to retain their certification,[45] such as:

- provision of evidence of staff qualifications, training, education and experience
- existence of an effective complaints process
- identification and traceability to ensure gametes, embryos and patients are correctly identified and matched at all times
- minimisation of the incidence of multiple pregnancy
- . . . and much more.

Australian National Health and Medical Research Council (NHMRC) *Ethical Guidelines*

In addition to the criteria contained in the RTAC *Code of Practice*, a set of guidelines, (outlined in a document titled the *Ethical guidelines on the use of assisted reproductive technology in clinical practice and research*) has been developed by the Australian National Health and Medical Research Council (NHMRC). As part of being certified/accredited, Australian fertility clinics are required to follow these guidelines.[46] The guidelines are subject to ongoing review.

The NHMRC *Ethical Guidelines on the use of assisted reproductive technology in clinical practice and research* provides a framework that works in conjunction with state, territory and Commonwealth legislation and governs all practitioners in their use of ART, [including fertility specialists (both independent or working as part of a clinic), nurses, embryologists, researchers, and so on] to ensure compliance with the guiding principles. These guiding principles include:

- the showing of respect to all involved
- consideration of the interests of donor-conceived children in the decision-making process
- harm minimisation
- the use of evidence-based practices
- transparency of practices
- the protection of people's privacy.[47]

At the heart of all ART legislation, codes of practice and ethical guidelines is the fundamental principle that the recipients of ART services and the children conceived remain the most important consideration in all decision-making processes.[48] While all of this is certainly a terrific exercise in responsibility and duty of care, it's important that the hordes of Australians seeking ART treatment are aware that Australia's fertility industry remains largely self-regulated.

What does self-regulation mean? It means that, rather than having an outside, independent agency monitor adherence to legal, ethical and safety standards, members of the industry complete these tasks themselves. For instance, at the time of writing, a significant majority of the FSANZ board members work at an Australian fertility clinic.[49]

Donor program

Irrespective of whether you are using a clinic-recruited donor or bringing your own known donor, the clinic will need to cater for the collection, testing process and storage of donor gametes and embryos. Not all clinics offer this service. In the case of embryo donation, it *might* be possible to move donated embryos from a clinic that does not offer an embryo donation program to one that can, assuming both of the donors and the embryo pass the requisite screening tests.

If you are considering an international donor, your Australian clinic needs to have a service agreement with an international sperm/egg bank. This comes with additional implications for you and, more importantly, for your child (see Chapter 8, 'Choosing an International Sperm/Egg Bank, or Egg Agency').

Public bank

Depending on where you live, you may have access to a public egg/sperm bank; embryo donation may also be available. Specific eligibility criteria will apply. For example, you may need to be a resident of the state or territory in which the egg/sperm bank is located, hold a Medicare card and be within a certain age range.

There may also be limitations imposed (such as a maximum number of cycles you can undergo) and, while the treatment itself may be free, you may incur some out-of-pocket expenses—such as for medication and diagnostic testing.

Processes and the way in which appointments are managed at public banks may also differ from the standard clinic approach. Check the local jurisdiction for more information about the rules and regulations applying to public banks in your location.

ART success rates

> *Facts are stubborn things, but statistics are pliable.*
>
> **Mark Twain**

Most clinics provide information about success rates on their websites and display data relevant to age and treatment type. Nevertheless, it is imperative you speak at length with the medical staff at your chosen clinic about their success rates and, more importantly, identify what those success rates actually *mean* and how they are *calculated.* For instance, does 'success' refer to the creation of an embryo suitable for transfer, or a positive pregnancy test, or are they referring to a baby that you can take home? Either way, be careful about using 'success rates' as your basis for choosing a clinic.[50]

Success rate variables

Success rates for fertility treatments are often inconsistent between clinics, largely because statistics depend on a number of different variables. Factors affecting data may include:

- the range of fertility treatments offered by the clinic
- the number of people included in the data
- whether people of forty years and over are restricted from accessing certain treatments
- how many embryos are transferred
- whether fresh or frozen embryos are transferred
- whether people are using frozen embryos created when the recipient was several years younger
- the possibility that success rates advertised by a smaller individual clinic *could* be based on data from its larger parent clinic.

Questions to ask at your clinic

When discussing the possibility of using donor conception to build your family, there are questions about success rates that you can ask at your clinic:

- Have you provided me with success rates relevant to my age?
- What is the difference in the success rates between using fresh embryos and using frozen embryos?
- Do you have access to the latest vitrification technology for successful frozen embryo transfers?

- Have you distinguished between live birth rates and clinical pregnancy rates (and mentioned that the live birth rate is the more meaningful statistic)?
- When was your success rate data collected?
- Is the data relevant for the type of treatment I will undergo (for example, IUI, IVF or ICSI)? (For more information about types of treatment see Chapter 11, 'Assisted Reproductive Technology [ART], "At-home" Insemination, Success Rates and Costs'.)
- Can you explain the factors that may impact my success rates, such as age, any previous pregnancies, lifestyle, etc.?

Whatever your situation, clinics are required to discuss the likelihood of you becoming pregnant via ART—and that discussion should be ongoing as you complete each treatment.[51] While statistics can provide a picture of what might occur, it is up to you to determine just how much influence the numbers have on your decision to proceed. Every clinic will supply you with data but, ultimately, the only success rate of consequence is the one that fits *your* personal circumstances.

IVF success estimator

To help Australians compare the (often confusing) clinic-advertised success rates more easily, the University of New South Wales, with the support of the Australian government, has set up a website called YourIVFSuccess.[52] The site provides information about IVF and helps you to locate a suitable clinic, as well as providing an interactive calculator to help you arrive at a basic estimate of your own conception chances.[53]

Choice of fertility specialists

> *I believe that choosing a fertility specialist is the single most important choice you will make throughout your entire fertility journey. If you make this decision in a calm and considered way, then you can sit back and trust that everything they are doing is in your best interests (not*

> *theirs!), and you can let them get on with doing what they are best at . . .*
>
> **Lucy Lines (Australian embryologist and contributing author to *Achieving parenthood*)**

The business of assisted reproduction does not generally align nicely with the business of a five-day working week and, while you might wish to have a specific doctor attend to *all* of your conception needs, it is possible—but it may not eventuate. Clinics are required to explain to you that a person other than your treating clinician may carry out certain procedures during the treatment process,[54] although they might neglect to mention this little detail.[55] So, if you don't wish to come face-to-face with a complete stranger when you arrive for a procedure, ensure you have an upfront discussion about who will be present at every step of the process.

Some people select a fertility specialist first and then the clinic is, subsequently, determined by that choice. Some specifically want a female specialist but, at a budget fertility clinic, you will usually see whoever is on duty on the day.

Staff experience and financial set-up

When selecting a fertility clinic, it may be worth considering the points discussed under the headings which follow.

Length of time the clinic has been operating

If the clinic has been operating for many years, you can be sure their website will announce this information quite clearly, probably on the Home page. The question to consider is, does it bother you if they've only been operating for a short period of time and, potentially, have limited success rate data collated?

If so, have a chat with the clinic to confirm the origins and background of their business. It is possible that, while being comparatively new, the clinic started with experienced staff who had come from another clinic. Just make sure you feel comfortable about the details before going ahead.

> ***Note:*** The NHMRC *Ethical Guidelines* require fertility clinics to disclose the level of experience of their staff.[56]

Experience and skill of the fertility specialist and the clinic's lab technicians

Is your fertility specialist 'a leader in the field'; an 'IVF pioneer'; or 'a member of the most highly-qualified team in the state' and possessed of 'unsurpassed experience'? Do they appear 'passionate about helping you to create a family'?[57]

Your specialist is the person who will assess your current situation and select an appropriate treatment plan for you. Is the specialist attentive? Do they listen to your needs and your partner's needs; and are they able to cater for these needs?

It is highly recommended you complete your own research to understand the options available to you and to ensure these align with your specialist's recommendations. Your specialist is also the person who will use their steady hands to transfer your blastocyst or embryo back into your body, or your partner's body. Research suggests that the skill and experience level of this specialist has an impact on success rates.[58]

The clinic's embryologists are the custodians of your precious gametes and embryos and the highest standards of quality control, teamwork and observational skills are required.[59] Again, your clinic must inform you of the experience level of your treating clinicians.[60]

Complete your homework and make an informed decision about whether you wish to go ahead with your chosen clinic and/or fertility specialist and their team members.

Financial set up of the clinic

To ensure patient safety and wellbeing are not compromised, Australian clinics are required to disclose any financial, personal or commercial interests which may be perceived as a conflict of interest relevant to the services or treatment they offer.[61]

Some questions you might wish to consider asking at your clinic include the following.

- Is it a family-owned clinic, or independently owned, or is it owned by staff who have a financial or commercial interest in the services provided?
- Do the fertility specialists operate independently of the clinic, or are they also employees?
- Does the clinic invest a percentage of income back into research in order to provide patients with the latest and greatest technology?
- Are there shareholders expecting dividends?
- Do the clinic or its shareholders invest any of their income into recruiting donors?

Choice of donors and selection process

> *We were given a spreadsheet of international sperm donors that our Queensland clinic had hand-picked from the US sperm bank's website. We went onto the sperm bank's website to check the profiles for ourselves and discovered the clinic had cut and pasted the features they wanted us to see. One donor on the clinic's list said he had olive skin, but they'd removed the bit that said he was actually Indian. Given we're both white, this might've impacted our child quite badly.*
>
> **Australian recipient parent**

Choice of donors

Sperm donors

The number of clinic-recruited sperm donors available at a clinic at any one time varies and can range from none to dozens of donors (sometimes waiting lists can be as long as twelve months). Several practices are registered Australia-wide and have clinics in more than one state or territory. Some of them may have a donor pool that all, or most, of their clinics can access. Other clinics may not have access to clinic-recruited donors at all and may only have capacity for you to bring your own known donor.

Your selection of sperm donors may be even further limited depending on what type of treatment you are undergoing—for example, IUI, IVF or ICSI (see Chapter 11, 'Assisted Reproductive Technology [ART], "At-home" Insemination, Success Rates and Costs').

Depending on the clinic and the number of donors available, you may be required to check for new donors on a daily basis because, when new donor profiles are uploaded, those donors can be snapped up within minutes.

Egg and embryo donors

Most clinics have an extremely long waiting list for their clinic-recruited egg and embryo donors—many have none available. Waiting lists can be as long as several years and intended parents are usually required to maintain regular contact to confirm their ongoing interest, otherwise they run the risk of being removed from the waiting list.

Often clinics don't even bother to offer the option of an egg or embryo donor and immediately direct intended parents to 'come back when you've found your own donor'.

Selection process

The way in which you select your donor—and the point at which the clinic provides access to the list of available donors—can vary significantly and may influence your choice of clinic. Following are some possible donor selection methods, but the list is not exhaustive.

Australian clinic-recruited sperm donor

***Option 1*:** You will be given the profiles of all available donors and asked to make a selection.

***Option 2*:** You will be provided with a couple of donor profiles from which to choose. Then, once you have eliminated one or both donors from your selection process, you will be provided with one or two further profiles, until you make a final decision. If you reject too many donors, you may be moved to the bottom of the waiting list.

***Option 3*:** You will be provided with a list of available donors that displays basic information, such as age, height, eye colour, and so on. Once you have shortlisted two or three potential donors, you will be given more detailed information about those donors to make your final choice.

***Option 4*:** You will be provided with two or three donor options and then, according to availability, will be advised (sometimes on the day of treatment) which donor you will be using.

Some clinics will limit the number of attempts you may have with a donor (for example, three) and then move you on to another donor if you don't conceive.

Australian clinic-recruited egg donor

In the unlikely event that one or more egg donors are available, you will be provided with the donors' profiles and be able to make a decision about whether you wish to go ahead with one of them.

International sperm and egg donors

The method by which you select your international donor can vary from clinic to clinic and alternative selection processes to those described below could be available. It is important to note that, just because your clinic offers the possibility of an international sperm or egg donor, it does not necessarily mean you get to trawl, carte blanche, through the bank's website and select the ultimate donor of your choice.

Following are some possible donor selection methods and related procedures.

1. In most cases, your Australian clinic will provide you with a list of donors from their affiliated sperm bank (or banks) who meet Australian regulatory and ethical standards, such as ID Release (see Chapter 16, 'ART Regulations and Ethical Guidelines'), and are available for the relevant treatment cycle you wish to undergo, for example, IUI or IVF (see Chapter 11, 'Assisted Reproductive Technology [ART], "At-home" Insemination, Success Rates and Costs'). In some cases, the clinic may direct you straight to the bank's website to make your selection from there.

2 Select a donor. You may be asked to select two or three donors, in order of preference, in case their gametes become unavailable between the time of your selection and payment. In the case of egg donation, the egg bank may provide you with two or three donors to choose from whose features match your own. You are able to reject these and ask for additional options but, usually, you cannot do this repeatedly.
   In the case of embryo donation (and, generally, in countries where donors are anonymous) the selection will often be made for you, usually attempting to match the physical features of you and/or your partner (see Chapter 8, 'Choosing an International Sperm/Egg Bank, or Egg Agency').
3 Pay for the number of sperm vials or eggs you wish to purchase. (In some cases there may not be a choice regarding how many you would like to purchase.) After payment, the gametes will be placed on hold for you.
4 The bank liaises with your Australian clinic and ships the gametes there in time for your treatment cycle. Alternatively, the Australian clinic may already have vials of sperm, pre-selected from the international sperm bank, in their freezer and ready for use.
5 If you are undergoing a double donation, with both an international sperm and egg donor, the gametes will usually be imported and fertilised at your Australian clinic.

If you wish to have a large selection of donors from which to choose, or you want a high degree of control over who your donor will be, it is definitely worth dedicating some time to identifying how individual clinics manage their donor selection process *before* you book an appointment. You might also like to view donor profiles on the banks' websites to ensure you are receiving the full (and correct) details.

> ***Note:*** Choosing an international donor comes with its own set of risks and should be considered carefully (see Chapter 8, 'Choosing an International Sperm/Egg Bank, or Egg Agency', and Chapter 9, Choosing Your Donor[s]').

Treatment eligibility

One of the first things you need to check at your chosen clinic is whether you are eligible for treatment there. Some clinics place restrictions on recipients when it comes to various aspects of the assisted reproduction process. For instance, some clinics may only offer fertility treatment with a donor if you live locally. Others have rigid guidelines concerning the age of the person seeking treatment.

If you are using a clinic-recruited sperm donor, you may find that some clinics restrict the number of times you can attempt IUI (for example, two attempts) before they move you on to IVF or ICSI. This is usually because IUI requires more samples from a donor and a subsequently greater time commitment, as well as high-quality sperm each time (see Chapter 11, 'Assisted Reproductive Technology [ART], "At-home" Insemination, Success Rates and Costs').

A 2020 Australian study[62] investigated why almost 60% of cisgendered lesbian, bisexual and queer (LBQ+) women underwent IVF, and suggested that clinics see IUI as a waste of sperm, as well as a waste of time and money for both the clinic and the patient. Some fertility specialists and staff who were interviewed as part of the study even suggested that, given the amount of money clinics receive from the government for an IVF cycle compared to an IUI cycle (1000% higher), profitability could be the driving force behind some clinics recommending IVF ahead of alternatives. One specialist went on to suggest that IUI success rates might appear lower than the reality due to the limited use of IUI by clinics.[63]

For people seeking embryo donation, clinics usually restrict the age of the recipients (this may be as low as forty, or as high as fifty years of age). Some clinics place a cap on an applicant's age at first application, but allow their age to exceed the cap while they wait for an embryo to become available. Clinics may also require an intended parent to have completed their own ART treatment prior to undergoing embryo donation—including having used all of their own frozen embryos in storage.

Waiting period

Waiting periods are usually dependent on two main factors. The first relates to the availability of doctors or fertility specialists. Some clinics claim to have a 'no wait' policy and guarantee an appointment within a certain number of days, while others make it clear that you will need to remain calm and breathe (or go elsewhere).

The second crucial factor is the availability of donors. While some of the larger operators may have a larger pool of sperm donors, you could be waiting months or even years for egg and embryo donors. Clinics affiliated with international banks usually have access to more donors.

Check with your prospective clinic about their waiting period before you make a commitment.

Personalised treatment

> *I ended up changing specialists because, after five failed IVF cycles with no embryos suitable for transfer, he said, 'Just keep going.'*
>
> **Australian intended parent**

Does the clinic offer customised treatment cycles, or is it a one-size-fits-all approach? Do they provide you with information and support regarding how best to prepare your body for pregnancy? Before ordering your fertility medication, if relevant, do they suggest undergoing diagnostic testing to check your reproductive system is in good working order? Do they explore all treatment options before recommending IVF or ICSI? Do they just keep saying, 'Let's do that again', even though 'that' isn't working?

Every person's body is different; one size does not fit all.

Clinic processes and procedures

Like all businesses, each clinic has its own way of doing things based on what they believe will provide the best outcomes for their customers—or is the most cost-effective, productive (and so on). It is definitely worth doing some research about fertility treatments to understand what the latest research indicates, and then to check your comfort levels about your chosen clinic's modus operandi.

Timing and location of treatment tests

During a treatment cycle, you may be required to undergo regular blood tests and ultrasounds to check the rate of egg growth and to ensure you are not suffering from ovarian hyperstimulation syndrome, (an exaggerated response to excess hormones). (See Chapter 13, 'Being a Donor and How it Works'.) Does your clinic provide the option of attending these tests in the morning so that you can still go to work? Are weekend appointments offered? If you choose a clinic in another state or territory, or in a city if you live regionally, can you undergo blood tests and ultrasounds locally then travel just for the main event? Or are you required to be physically present at the clinic for every step of the process?

Availability of advanced technology and 'add-ons'

> *While I was happy to do some testing because of my age, the clinic wanted to test everything in sight. I had to push back and trust in the process.*
>
> **Australian recipient parent**

Fertility clinics are heavily invested in helping you achieve your pregnancy goals and technology is advancing all the time. Most clinics offer supplementary treatments and services, otherwise known as 'adjuvant treatments', 'adjunct treatments' or 'add-ons'. Add-on procedures include: ovarian rejuvenation; endometrial scratching; and more. Add-ons often incur additional costs, ranging from a few dollars to several thousands of dollars (although a clinic *might* include a 'complimentary' add-on as part of a treatment). The add-ons are not usually covered by Medicare or private health insurance.

Despite the expense of add-ons, many people use them in the hope of increasing their chances of achieving a pregnancy— some people *insist* that a particular add-on be used.

But are add-ons actually worth it? When deciding on any method or the use of technology, particularly when medication or surgery is involved, it's important to identify whether the technology is evidence-based. In other words, will the add-on treatment potentially increase your chances of conception and reduce your risk of miscarriage or, conversely, is there a possibility that it may even do you or your embryo harm? A 2021 study investigated twenty-one different add-ons advertised on multiple Australasian fertility clinic websites and concluded that none of those add-ons were supported by 'high-quality evidence' that resulted in improved rates of pregnancy or live births.[64] A 2023 study examining twenty-seven add-ons also indicated that none of the success claimed for those add-ons could be based on high-quality-evidence and only four could provide 'moderate-quality evidence'. Some add-ons demonstrated no beneficial effects or lacked a correct theoretical foundation, while others even raised serious safety concerns.[65]

New technology is constantly emerging so, if you are undergoing ART treatment at a clinic, ensure your specialist provides you with a list of the available add-ons, including a clear explanation that each *is* an add-on and not standard protocol, and accurate information about each option, including evidence of its effectiveness, its risks and the costs involved.[66] Then you can make an informed decision about whether you wish to proceed, or not.

Costs and payment options

All clinics must provide intended parents with information about the likely fees and out-of-pocket expenses so that they can make an informed financial decision.[67] It is definitely worth shopping around— the same treatment can vary significantly between clinics. And remember that cheaper is not always better.

It is also important to note that sometimes it's not actually possible to compare 'apples with apples' when costs such as 'donor management fee', which may cover a range of different items depending on the clinic, appears on your invoice.

Bulk-billing options

Some Australian clinics offer bulk-billing options for some of their procedures, but specific eligibility criteria might apply.

In all cases, check with the clinic to determine whether they cut any sizeable corners that may, or may not, suit your requirements.

- Are you able to select a specific doctor?
- Is the treatment offered a standard, inflexible protocol using minimal medication, or can it be tailored to suit your needs?
- What are their success rates?
- Are only certain donor types available? For example, does bulk-billing still apply if you bring your own known donor to the clinic?

Paying for gametes

When paying a clinic for your donor's sperm, one aspect you need to be aware of is the point at which you will be asked to hand over your money. Do you need to pay for it as soon as you've selected your donor, or can you wait until you're ready to undergo ART treatment? Will the clinic let you purchase just one vial, or do they insist on you buying several?

Of course, there are pros and cons to this quandary. For instance, if you are unsuccessful on your first treatment cycle and you wish to purchase more vials, there may be none remaining or your selected donor may be unavailable. Furthermore, if you wish to have more than one child using the same donor, it may be beneficial to purchase more than one vial and store the sperm in the clinic's freezer.

In many cases, clinics will put aside another vial for you if you do become pregnant but have indicated you'd like another child in the future.

Egg donation is usually charged at a set fee and eggs retrieved during the donor's cycle are included as part of the treatment.

If you are using frozen, imported donor gametes, you will generally be required to pay for those upfront (see Chapter 8, 'Choosing an International Sperm/Egg Bank, or Egg Agency').

Payment options

Some clinics offer different payment options, such as a 'no upfront fee' payment plan for Medicare-eligible patients. This means you don't need to pay anything until a certain point in the process, so you'll be out-of-pocket for a shorter period of time than you would otherwise have been. In certain circumstances, it is also possible to access your superannuation to fund fertility treatment, but an approval process is required.

Some other payment options offered by various fertility clinics include:

- bulk billing of your initial appointment (prior to making decisions about treatment)
- free fertility assessment
- part-payment upfront, with the balance paid at a later date
- payment instalment plans
- price reduction once a certain number of cycles have been completed within one year
- concession pricing (for example, Health Care Card holders)
- concession pricing for rural and remote patients
- applications for financial assistance in cases of financial hardship
- complimentary storage for frozen eggs, sperm and embryos for one year (or other specified time period).

Screening

For more information on donor screening see Chapter 13, 'Being a Donor and How it Works'.

Location

Various factors might influence the location of the clinic you select, including your preferred fertility specialist, availability (or location) of donors, treatment options, the clinic itself, and so on.

While travel may seem like a great option for you (or, if applicable, your known donor), there are several aspects to consider.

Cost

Can you afford to travel to undergo ART treatment, with the possibility of further treatments at the same location in the future? Some of the costs involved include flights, accommodation, car hire, parking, meals and time off work.

Embryos

If you create embryos and wish to undergo further treatment or to have another child, what are the processes, risks and costs involved in importing your embryos back to your state or territory? Alternatively, will you need to keep returning to the location where your embryos are stored?

Access to donor and siblings

Many donor-conceived people tell us that having contact (or, at least, having the choice) with siblings and the donor is vital (see Chapter 15, 'Donor and Sibling Linking'). At what stage would you like this to occur for your donor-conceived child and how will you manage connections if the donor lives on the other side of the country and siblings are spread far and wide?

Communication

> *Yesterday I had my third egg retrieval. Today I had a phone appointment with my fertility specialist to discuss the results from my second round, and yesterday's results. He started the conversation by saying the results from the second round*

aren't back yet. I corrected him and told him I got the results about a week ago. He asked me to talk him through them, and then he said he didn't have yesterday's results yet. I told him the nurse called me a few hours ago with the results and that he will be able to see them in the system. We then discussed when I should do the transfer. He said I should discuss this with my partner and he thinks it would be better to take a month off to bond with my partner, spend time cuddling and rekindle the relationship before next steps. I reminded him that I'm single. This specialist is head of the medical board at the clinic. He is supposed to be an amazing doctor.

Australian recipient parent

When deciding which clinic or specialist to use, remember that although the clinic may appear to be offering you a solution to all of your problems and, no doubt many of the staff will have your best interests at heart, they are still a business invested in making money. A 2019 inquiry into Victorian ART practices indicated that, in many cases, communication was either poorly delivered or ineffective and made it difficult for people to make informed decisions.[68] As two different Australian parents explained to me, experiences vary enormously and can range from:

I had a really good experience at my clinic. The specialist was really supportive, especially after multiple failed cycles, and encouraged me to take rests in between cycles.

to:

Our clinic was so bad at returning calls that I had to leave a message on their Instagram account saying, 'I've got cash and I want to use you,' in order to get them to call me.

How do you rate your clinic's communication?

Do your research, talk to others who have used their services, make a list of your own questions and ring or email the clinic to discuss them;

and, if they exist, locate online forums to view other families' opinions, and attend free fertility seminars the clinic might run.

Get a second opinion, if necessary, then make an informed decision. Of course, everyone has different preferences and needs: what you're looking for may be quite different to someone else's version of excellence so, perhaps the most important aspect to consider about your clinic or your specialist is what feels right for *you*.

Ethics

While there are many outstanding specialists and staff to be found in Australian clinics, and stories of excellent service abound, the 2019 enquiry into ART practices (referred to earlier) indicated that poor behaviour is also evident.[69] If you have started doing your own research through social media groups, you may have come across rumours about fertility specialists who cut corners; or hyperstimulation of egg donors (184 people across Australia and New Zealand were admitted to hospital in 2019 with ovarian hyperstimulation syndrome[70]); or those who suggest that, instead of using a sperm donor: 'Why not go down to the local pub and find yourself a good-looking bloke and have a one-night stand?' (Yes, there are many reports of this.)

If a specialist, or any other staff member at a clinic, exhibits any behaviours that don't feel 'right' to you, ensure you make a complaint (if warranted), choose another specialist and, possibly, another clinic.

Complaint process

If you feel you are being discriminated against or treated unfairly at your chosen clinic, file a complaint. Clinics are required to have a policy for investigation and resolution of complaints,[71] although some have been known to neglect any mention of its existence to their patients.[72]

If you do not feel satisfied with the outcome of your complaint, you can escalate it to the Reproductive Technology Accreditation Committee (RTAC), the Australian Competition and Consumer Commission (ACCC), the Office of Fair Trading in your state or territory, or the Health Complaints Commission (or equivalent) if one exists in your state or territory. If your issue is about an individual health practitioner whom you believe to be placing the public at risk, practising their profession in an unsafe way, or making unsafe judgments due to ill health, you can report your complaint to the Australian Health Practitioner Regulation Agency (APHRA).

> **Note:** So that the RTAC can monitor complaints, a clinic is required to advise the Chair of the RTAC if a complaint notification about one of their practitioners is received from the ACCC, APHRA or the Department of Fair Trading.[73]

In rare cases involving extreme circumstances, such as a clinic using the wrong donor, the only way forward might be to employ your own legal team if the regulatory organisations are unwilling or unable to assist you.

Support process

> *I was really upset by the lack of support from my clinic when I had a miscarriage. All I got from them was, 'When would you like to come back?'*
>
> **Australian intended parent**

There is no question that undergoing fertility treatment involves some big emotional responses. Add donor conception to the equation and feelings can escalate even further. What if you need help throughout the treatment process, or during pregnancy? What if you are experiencing multiple failed cycles, unsuccessful pregnancies, or you're feeling depressed after you've given birth?

All clinics provide counsellors for pre-treatment counselling and these counsellors can also be used at any time throughout your treatment or pregnancy (although reports suggest gaining access to those counsellors can be difficult).[74] If you don't feel comfortable using the clinic's counsellor, or they are not available, you can use your own. There are also many, many support groups available. Some clinics run their own support programs and claim to provide high quality assistance to help patients through any personal issues related to infertility, conception and pregnancy.

Make sure you inform yourself about what's available to you (or ask a friend or loved one to help if you don't have the capacity to inform yourself), and don't be afraid to seek help if you need it. (See 'Useful tools and resources' at the back of this book for links to online sources containing additional resources, blog articles and the latest updates, including information about available support.)

8

Choosing an International Sperm/Egg Bank, or Egg Agency

When we try to advocate for change as donor-conceived people, we are up against the multinational corporations with their millions of dollars and professional lawyers. We are constantly trying to raise awareness about the rights of the child, but we can't do this alone—fertility clinics only exist because of their clients and you have a right to demand changes when you see and hear about unethical practices, because you are the paying client!

Australian donor-conceived adult (Vic.)

Note: Ensure you have read Chapter 7, 'Choosing an Australian Fertility Clinic', before reading this chapter.

If you are considering using an international donor, the two biggest questions to consider are, how will that impact you and, more importantly, how will that impact your *child*?

Has your Australian clinic suggested 'international is best' before you've even stepped over the threshold? Do you feel exhilarated by the sheer volume of donors to choose from: a veritable deluge of good-looking adults, all willing to hand over their gametes for a pretty sum?

For some people, finding a local Australian donor is not easy—for others, it's impossible. For instance, donors of certain races and ethnicity are frequently hard to come by, as are donors who have been screened to avoid specific inherited diseases (although additional screening can usually be requested).

Choosing a donor from another country involves a substantial amount of research and an even greater deal of consideration. If you do decide to go ahead with an international donor, which country and which international sperm/egg bank or clinic/agency should you choose? All countries have significantly different policies, processes, ethical standards and legislation from Australia. There are many factors you need to consider.

Accreditation and standards

> *I created a Facebook group and actively look for other families. We are in contact with six so far. They have all reported different numbers supplied to them by the US sperm bank—one mother was told over five, another was told less than five. On the same day.*
>
> **Australian recipient parent**

Around the globe, the fertility industry is expanding and evolving all the time—and many argue that these changes are not for the better. Nevertheless, donors are in demand right now and banks and agencies are constantly updating their customer options and improving the professional look and feel of their websites. Banks are screening for more diseases, adding more variables to help intended parents narrow down their selection, constantly introducing more technology—'thumbs up' to move Donor A99 to your Favourites list; 'thumbs down' to delete Donor F11—and so on.

Dozens of countries are catering for sperm, egg and embryo donation—donors short and tall (although mostly tall); young and attractive; brown-eyed or blue-eyed; fair haired or dark (usually not red). Each country has different laws, different regulations (or no regulations), different standards and, in some countries (Australia included), the legislation varies between states, territories, counties or provinces. For instance, some countries have a complete ban on all forms of treatment in which donors are used, while others allow donor sperm for heterosexual married couples only. Some countries impose strict limits on: the number of embryos transferred (while others have no limits); the number of families that can use a donor; and the storage limits of frozen embryos (while some countries don't allow embryos to be frozen at all). In some countries, all donors are anonymous, while in others (including Australia) anonymity is banned. Some countries consider it acceptable to give excess frozen embryos away without permission from the owners.

> *. . . people should think about fertility doctors like they do used car dealers.*
>
> **Jim Hawkins (Professor of Law at the University of Houston, USA)**[75]

If you decide to use an international donor, either through an Australian clinic or by travelling to a foreign country, it is important to check the standards that apply in the relevant country and whether these standards are actually enforced. For example, a US sperm bank's website might display their recommended family limits, but there may be no legislation in place to impose these limits; so the sperm bank can change them or ignore them, at will—and some have done just that.

If you are considering choosing an international donor via your Australian clinic, don't assume the standards of the relevant country are either ethical, or considered.

International donor program

If you are choosing an international donor through your Australian clinic, the origins of your donor will be dictated by your Australian clinic's affiliated bank or agency. Some have service agreements with banks in multiple countries, while others have none. Some international banks also import gametes from *other* countries or, alternatively, they use gametes from people who are not permanent residents but are currently residing or studying there. This fact may not necessarily be disclosed on donors' profiles—check with the bank or agency if you're not sure.

If you are travelling to a foreign country for part or all of your treatment, the choice of countries—as well as the risks—increase considerably.

Success rates

While Australia has standards in place related to the advertising of ART success rates and this is monitored by independent bodies such as the ACCC, does your international bank or agency have similar standards? Is there any legislation or policy in place to ensure you are being provided with accurate data? Is the data based on pregnancies or live births? Is it relevant to your circumstances?

The questions above are just some you may wish to ask your clinic or agency. (For more information about success rates see Chapter 7, 'Choosing an Australian Fertility Clinic').

Choice of fertility specialists

If you are travelling overseas to undergo ART treatment and wish to use a particular fertility specialist, you may need to check with the relevant clinic that this is actually possible. If it is, ensure that your travel plans align with the specialist's timetable. Depending on the location and size of the clinic, there may only *be* one specialist.

Staff experience and financial structure

In a similar manner to Australian clinics, it is worth investigating your international bank or agency and the staff with whom you will be working. How long has the clinic been operating? Is the staff (fertility specialists, embryologists, etc.) appropriately qualified? Has the bank recently been taken over by a larger corporation? (This could impact multiple aspects of your experience, including the extent to which your donor is screened and the number of siblings your donor-conceived child ends up with.)

Choice of donors and selection process

The following information is relevant to people who travel to a foreign country to select a donor. For information about choosing an international donor via an Australian clinic, see Chapter 7, 'Choosing an Australian Fertility Clinic'.

Sperm and egg donors

International sperm and egg donors are usually in abundant supply (especially when they are paid). The donor selection process varies depending on the country. When donors are featured on a website, there tends to be a generous amount of information and, in some cases, adult photos may be available.

Your choice of donors will be influenced by their availability. For instance, if your chosen egg donor has a personal commitment at the time you wish to travel, you will need to find a different donor—or wait. The same thing applies if the vials of sperm from your selected sperm donor have run out. Sometimes, after selecting two or three donor options, the process of confirming your final donor may take several weeks of 'toing and froing'.

Alternatively, particularly in countries where anonymity is the only option, the clinic may choose your donor for you and you might receive very limited information about the donor. Their selection will usually be based on the phenotypic information that you provide about yourself and your partner (obvious observable traits, such as hair colour), as well as other important factors, such as blood group and genetic testing. The clinic may even claim to have fancy technology that matches you and your donor via a facial resemblance system. In some countries, it may even be legislated that your donor needs to look as similar to you as possible.

Embryo donation

If you are undergoing embryo donation in a foreign country, your embryo donors may be anonymous. Depending on the country, embryos might be sourced from people who have excess embryos following IVF, or created using the agency's own sperm and egg donors. In many cases, the agency will select the embryos for you and there will be an attempt to match your features with those of the embryo donors (as per the previous section on 'Sperm and egg donors').

Double donation

If you are undergoing double donation in a foreign country, after choosing your egg donor you may be able to select a sperm donor from the international sperm bank of your choice and have the sperm shipped to your chosen country's clinic, or you may need to select a sperm donor who is local to the country in which you are undergoing treatment. If you are required to select from the relevant country's list of sperm donors, check whether they have an 'anonymous only' rule (see Chapter 16, 'ART Regulations and Ethical Guidelines'). If you select an anonymous donor and need to undergo a frozen embryo transfer (FET) cycle at a later date (see Chapter 11, 'Assisted Reproductive Technology [ART], "At-home" Insemination, Success Rates and Costs'), you will not be able to ship the embryos back to an Australian clinic but will need to return to the relevant country to complete the cycles there.

Furthermore, if you choose to import sperm to your chosen country for a double donation, some countries require you to obtain an import permit, which may take up to several weeks (or even months). You should be able to track the permit's progress around the globe from your computer. Depending on the country and the clinic, they may assist you with this process, or even obtain the permit on your behalf.

Once you have the permit, you can import the sperm, which might take a further few weeks to arrive. If your cycle is unsuccessful, you will have to repeat the whole process again, so obtaining more than one vial of sperm is potentially a good idea.

The importation of sperm to the country in which you are undergoing treatment can be an extremely expensive exercise.

In all cases, when deciding which path to choose, it is important to consider the needs of your donor-conceived child.

Treatment eligibility

If you are undergoing ART treatment in a foreign country, you will be restricted by the policies within that country. For instance, some countries only allow heterosexual married couples to use donor gametes or embryos, while others may have strict policies related to age. Some have different rules in place for sperm, egg and embryo donations. In countries where donors are paid, where large quantities of gametes are collected and you are handing over large amounts of cash, it is likely you will be eligible for most treatment options.

Clinic processes and procedures

> *There was absolutely nothing sub-standard about the clinic I attended overseas. The testing and the medical assessments I had to undergo were incredibly thorough. The fertility specialist was great and the whole experience was excellent. There was even an Australian nurse over there.*
>
> **Australian recipient parent**

Processes and procedures vary significantly between countries and clinics—including standards of care and safety. Some people report extremely positive experiences and high standards of care; others have terrible ordeals. Some of these include:

- inadequate donor screening resulting in life-threatening diseases for the children who are born
- concerns about the qualification and skills of the specialist
- having the door opened with regularity while being examined and being exposed to whoever is walking past
- rough and painful internal examinations
- a lack of formal appointment times and, instead, waiting for hours to be squeezed in between local patients' appointments
- an inability to communicate effectively and understand local protocols.

In some countries, donor conception is impacted by legislation, or lack thereof. Sometimes it is influenced by politics and religion. In all cases, make sure you check the ART treatment protocols in the country of your choice and ensure they favourably compare with Australian industry standards.

> ***Note:*** In countries where policy and legislation does not align with Australia's—including donor anonymity—it will not be possible to import any excess embryos back into Australia. This means you will need to travel to the relevant country to undergo further attempts at conception with your frozen embryos (see Chapter 16, 'ART Regulations and Ethical Guidelines').

Availability of advanced technology

Sometimes international clinics claim to have more advanced technology than is available in Australia. In all scenarios, ensure you carry out appropriate research and establish whether the technology in question may actually help, or whether it could potentially cause harm. (For more information about add-ons see Chapter 7, 'Choosing an Australian Fertility Clinic'.)

Costs and payment options

The cost of ART treatment varies *significantly* between countries. If you are tempted to make decisions based on financial considerations you may come to regret later, remember that some overseas clinics, while offering lower prices, also have poor standards and this is likely to affect all areas of medical care.

Paying for flights, accommodation, meals and local transport in your country of choice can also add thousands of dollars to your fertility experience, particularly if you need to make multiple trips to use all of your embryos. Some clinics in certain countries offer a package deal in which they take care of everything you will need in that country. This might include booking your accommodation for you, arranging travel from the airport and daily travel to and from the clinic, and so on. It may also include extras such as acupuncture or massage—these packages, of course, do come at a cost in addition to the cost of your ART treatment.

Travel

One important aspect to consider when choosing fertility treatment overseas is the travel involved. How far away is your chosen country? How frequent are flights and how much do they cost? Will the duration of the flight, including stopovers, along with the subsequent time it takes to arrive at your final destination impact the number of days leave you need to take? Does your partner need to travel as well to provide gametes for the embryo you are creating?

If you are travelling to a foreign country to undergo a fresh transfer with an egg donor, your egg donor may also be required to travel. For instance, is the donor local to the clinic where the ART treatment will take place, or do they live on the other side of the country? If it is the latter situation, you will also be paying your donor's travel and accommodation costs, potentially adding thousands of dollars to your final bill.

Ensure your travel insurance covers you for fertility treatment overseas in case of unforeseen events such as ovarian hyperstimulation syndrome, infection or other complications.

Paying for gametes and treatment

When it comes to paying for gametes, some international sperm banks place a minimum limit on the number of vials that can be purchased. This might be as few as two vials, or as many as ten. If you don't wish to purchase that many vials, you may need to consider a different sperm bank and, ergo, a different clinic. The timing of your payments will depend on the local policies and, while you may be able to pay in instalments as the process unfolds (for example, donor selection, then egg collection), in most cases, you will be required to pay the entire balance of your treatment *before* you leave Australia.

Different countries offer different methods of paying for your gametes and ART treatment, as well as for additional expenses such as medication. These methods might include international transfers or credit card payments. Do your homework on your chosen country and ensure your method of payment is not high risk for fraud.

It might also be a good idea to let your bank or other financial institution know before you make any overseas transactions, so they don't assume you are being scammed and leave you without cash for an extended period of time. Some countries prefer (and even encourage) you to pay in cash and will give you a discount if you are willing to receive a receipt for an amount less than the actual price paid—consider carefully whether this reflects on their overall standards.

Screening

> *We travelled overseas because we wanted to find a donor with the same ethnicity as my husband, and also because it was significantly cheaper than Australia. My daughter now has a rare disease where she is in constant pain. I can't begin to tell you how much I regret our decision to go to a country with poor screening and medical practices—seeing my child suffer is like a form of torture.*
>
> **Australian recipient parent**

While it is not possible to screen for everything, simply because there are unknown diseases for which we don't yet have a test, it's good to know exactly which screening tests your donor *has* undergone. For instance, have they been tested for basic health issues only (such as sexually transmitted diseases), or have they also completed a comprehensive set of genetic tests? The clinic or bank's website will usually list the screening tests undertaken, or you can call them to discuss this.

In some countries fairly limited genetic testing is completed on donors while, in others, extensive screening is carried out and additional (paid) tests for specific diseases or disorders are also provided on request. This may be helpful if you are a carrier of a disease and need to select a different donor.

The way in which your donor is screened can have serious long-term impacts on the health of your child, as well as on your child's children. Be aware that mistakes and oversights have been made in the past and continue to be made today.

Counselling

> *Donor counselling should be mandatory with an independent third party so parents really understand what they're getting themselves into. Creating a child isn't something that should be undertaken lightly. It's a decision that will affect the rest of your life, and the lives of many other people too.*
>
> **Australian donor-conceived adult (NSW)**

If you are using an international donor via an Australian clinic, donors are required to be counselled to Australian standards. However, if you are travelling to another country to undergo ART treatment, the same may not be true.

Do you know the guidelines in your chosen country? Sometimes the counselling can be excellent; one Australian recipient parent describes their experience as follows:

> *The international clinic I attended had compulsory counselling. I didn't realise this is quite rare. It had to be done face-to-face and covered lots of important issues, most of which I'd already researched but I was impressed all the same.*

In other countries, donors are not required to undergo any counselling at all and may have little or no understanding of the number of children they may be about to bring forth into the world—and no information about the rights and needs of donor-conceived people. This may have serious consequences for your child if they attempt to contact the donor at a later date, or when your child finds out they have one hundred siblings scattered around the globe.

Regulation and policy

> *Do you* [people who work in the fertility industry] *ever consider that the humans you help create might be curious, family-oriented people who may want to know their origin*

> *story and all of the family who hold a place in their DNA? These people are in fact bits of you. Their DNA, their very essence, is our own. Our biological family impacts who we are in profound ways, from physical appearance, to likes and dislikes, to physical and mental health. Is that ever a thought that comes to mind in your line of work?*
>
> **Donor-conceived teenager (13 years old)**

Although Australian clinics might have a service agreement in place with their international affiliated sperm or egg banks to ensure they align with Australian standards, displaying some healthy scepticism in this area will not go to waste. Make sure you quiz your chosen clinic about their affiliated sperm or egg bank—and then cross-examine the international bank directly with the same set of questions. But be warned, it is still possible you may not get to the truth of the matter (see 'Ethics' later in this chapter).

Alternatively, if you are travelling to a foreign country to undergo ART treatment, it's vital to understand that Australian laws and medical standards do not apply and you may not be protected if something goes wrong.

Some issues for you to consider when making your decisions about an international donor and the relevant country's sperm or egg bank/ agency are discussed under the following headings.

Regulation and guidelines

- What are the current ART regulations and guidelines in that country (if any) and what implications might they have for you, your donor and, more importantly, your donor-conceived child?
- What kind of documentation are you required to sign? Is it worth having the documents reviewed by an Australian lawyer?
- What are the regulations and policies related to medical standards? For instance, sometimes practices considered to be high risk in Australia (for example, multiple embryo transfers) are more frequently accepted in other countries.

Processes and procedures

- What success rates do they advertise? Can the numbers be validated?
- What are the criteria for donor selection? What are the age limits, and is medical history and residency status recorded?
- How extensive are the medical and genetic screening processes? Can you pay to have additional screening tests upon request?
- Are criminal background checks conducted on their donors?
- What are their worldwide family limits? How do they track them, if at all? Does the bank or agency follow up with its recipients, or is the onus on the recipient parents to report a live birth? (See 'Family limits and siblings' in Chapter 9, 'Choosing your donor'.)

Recordkeeping

> *Fires and floods at clinics are a common story, so much so that it has become a running joke in the donor-conceived community.*
>
> **Australian donor-conceived adult (NSW)**

How effective are your bank or agency's recordkeeping policies? Do they maintain contact with your donor? Do they ask the donor to notify the bank or agency should any known medical issues arise with them or their family? Or, do they collect data when the donor provides their gametes and then never contact them again?

It's also interesting to note that, in some cases, banks won't *allow* you to report a live birth if you have used an on-donated embryo, because you are not the original recipient of the gametes.

How long is your bank or agency required to keep records? Does legislation related to data collection and maintenance exist, or are there only recommendations? What about company closure or takeover? Do you trust that your records will be handed over to the new company? Will your records be housed in a government archiving centre in a suburban backwater—impossible to locate? Or will they become 'lost' in a flood or a fire, two natural disasters that seem to occur frequently when donor-conceived people seek information about their conception?

Travelling with medication

If you travel to another country to undergo ART treatment, you may be required to bring medication and syringes home with you. In this instance, ask the local fertility clinic to provide you with a letter of authorisation so you can get them through customs without any problems arising.

Complaint process

If you are using an international donor via an Australian clinic, then all of the Australian complaint processes apply (see Chapter 7, 'Choosing an Australian Fertility Clinic'). If you have a problem with the international sperm or egg bank you use, you can try contacting them directly—however it may prove challenging to procure the information you're seeking.

If you are travelling overseas to undergo ART treatment, you will be at the mercy of the local clinic and that country's processes and ethical standards (or lack thereof).

Anonymity versus Open ID

> *We chose anonymous because that's all they offered in the country we went to and because it was cheaper. We were both ignorant of the consequences of choosing an anonymous donor and how it would affect our child's life. Looking back, I would choose an open donor. Now it's too late and we can't turn back time.*
>
> **Australian recipient parent**

In some countries, the law requires donors to be anonymous; in others it is simply the clinic's policy and can vary between clinics. Some international agencies, banks and clinics are open to the option of asking the donor if they would be willing to be known. This may also happen in 'anonymous only' countries where discussions about possible changes to the legislation are occurring.

Some clinics will even provide you with snippets of information about the donor, or you might see the donor walk into their appointment with the specialist directly after yours. Sometimes anonymous donors make requests of the bank to change their 'anonymous' status to 'known'. There is, of course, no guarantee that the bank will agree to this; that the legislation will change; or that the donor, should they choose this option, will honour the decision. Holding out for these possibilities is a risky enterprise and your child is the one who will suffer any negative consequences. An Australian embryo recipient describes her experience:

> *I asked my international egg donor if she would be open to contact and she said yes. After my daughter was born, I sent a letter of thanks to the clinic to pass on and I haven't heard anything back several years later.*

If you are undergoing anonymous embryo donation, there is a possibility the clinic has shared any excess embryos with multiple families. This means your child will have full siblings located around the world, with limited or no means of identifying them and connecting. There may also be half siblings if egg and/or sperm donors were used to create the embryo.

If a bank or agency decides to change the existing policy regarding anonymity in the future, they may insist you complete a new contract and charge you for them to reveal your donor's identity. Given they will already have this information on file somewhere, a request for more funds in this situation could reasonably be considered unethical.

Some international clinics will facilitate a known donation if the request is made via an agency, or an intended parent might arrange it independently. Some people plan to DNA test their child in order to find their anonymous donor. However, there are many countries that do not do a significant amount of testing—in some countries it is banned—so, finding people in these countries can be difficult, if not impossible (see Chapter 15, 'Donor and Sibling Linking').

Communication

> *My mum died suddenly from an aneurysm related to a genetic disease that she passed to half of her children, five years AFTER I donated my eggs. I immediately had testing and notified the clinic where I donated. That was in 2005. They never contacted the recipients' families. I've since found five of the seven young adults conceived from my eggs and one has the disease at this stage. Despite reaching out to the clinic again in 2017, they still haven't contacted any of these families.*
>
> **American egg donor**

Communication is a vital consideration when selecting an international donor and, in the case of extreme medical issues such as inherited disease, may be the difference between your child's life and death. Following are some issues to consider when making your decision about an international donor and the relevant country's bank or agency.

- If you are travelling to a foreign country to undergo an ART procedure, do the staff at the relevant clinic speak English (or your first language)? If not, will your Australian clinic communicate with them on your behalf? Can you be certain that your requirements will be understood and met? Is there an interpreter available to ensure you understand protocols? Are they familiar with Australians, Australian requirements, and so on?
- Have they reviewed your file before you enter their rooms? Do they have an understanding of your medical history? Do they even know who you are, or do you have to explain your situation repeatedly?
- Do they seem organised, or is the whole process in the foreign clinic chaotic and unsettling?
- Do they treat you like they would a local patient, or do you feel like an unwanted intruder?
- Do they keep switching donors on you?
- Do they object when you ask for a copy of the contract?

- Do you have to liaise with multiple parties (clinic, agency, bank, etc.)? Is the process complicated and stressful?
- Do they cancel appointments without telling you?
- Do they respond quickly to your emails or calls (or other form of communication), or are you left anxious and fearful that you will lose your donor because you haven't locked in the agreement and paid within the requisite time? Time zone differences can produce significant delays in responses, which may create challenges when making arrangements.
- Do they inform you about the quality of the embryos and how many they are transferring, or do they just go ahead with the procedure without informing you?
- Do they follow up with you if you have an unsuccessful embryo transfer or a miscarriage?
- What communication options do they offer once your child is born? For example, do they have a voluntary register where you can communicate with other families who have used the same donor—and where siblings can connect with each other, as well as with the donor?
- Do they have an effective policy in place for maintaining contact with their donors so they can pass on important medical information and provide your child with up-to-date identifying information when they turn eighteen (or another specified age)? Furthermore, are they willing to contact the *donor* about health issues should they arise in your child/children, so the donor can protect their own children? Or does the information only go one way?
- How will they contact you should any health issues arise with your donor at a later date? Do they have a history of *not* sharing information or not informing relevant parties about donor or children's health issues? In rare cases, the strength of this policy—and subsequent action—may save your child's life.
- When you ask, will they disclose the number of siblings your child has?
- Where there is no donor register, will they pass on your request for contact with the donor?

Ethics

> *In the end,* [Justice] *Nahmias summed up the debate asking, 'just to be clear, what you're asserting, a sperm bank can completely misrepresent everything about the sperm itself and charge whatever amount of money based on those representations and completely lie to every customer it has—and nobody can do a thing about it?'*
>
> **Justice David Nahmias**
> **(quoted from a case before the Supreme Court of Georgia, USA)**[76]

The US sperm bank's response to the question posed by Justice Nahmias was: 'Under the law, yes'. The sperm bank referred to in the quote is used by multiple Australian clinics.

While there are many success stories, the international donor conception industry is riddled with stories of lies and deception.[77] Before you choose an international donor—be it via your Australian clinic, or by way of an expedition to the southern tip of Africa—it's important to understand what you're getting into.

Donor exploitation

An important question you need to ask is, how are donors sourced in the country you select? For instance, are the young sperm donors (eighteen and nineteen year olds in some instances) lured by the promise of enduring pocket money for the term of their college experience? Do they have any understanding of the lasting effects of their regular long-term contributions at the local sperm bank? Are they aware that each donation is probably being separated into multiple sperm vials each time and then sold for multiple years to multiple families?

In the case of egg donors, do you know whether your donor has been sourced from an impoverished country, offered meagre remuneration and then dangerously hyperstimulated to produce large numbers of children and maximum profit? Is the donor providing their eggs to one family per cycle, or are their eggs being distributed to multiple families, resulting in large sibling groups? Do the donors receive a finder's fee for recruiting their friends, which helps perpetuate the sale of anonymous gametes? If your donor's gametes are of poor quality, has anyone made your donor aware of this fact? Do these donors undergo counselling to help them understand the lasting effects of their actions and the needs of the donor-conceived people they're helping to create?

Alternatively, are you aware that you could be seeking an embryo in a country where women who no longer have male partners can be forced into giving up their excess embryos to couples wanting an embryo?[78]

In countries around the world right now, all of these scenarios are happening. It is up to intended parents to bring about change by seeking alternative options, to make more informed, ethical choices to stop the exploitation of vulnerable people for the sake of profit margins and to avoid the potential trauma experienced by the donor-conceived children being created.

Contracts

> *This is what is wrong with the donor conception industry: the expectation that two parties—i.e. the donor and recipient—can make a binding agreement for an absent third party—i.e. the child. That expectation is being challenged by donor-conceived individuals and groups.*
>
> **Australian recipient parent**

Depending on how you access a donor, you may have to sign a contract. If you do, ensure that you read the fine print. Take it a step further and ask to view a sample copy of the bank's *donor* contract, just in case it contains clauses you feel are unethical. For example, in the past, some US sperm banks required donor-conceived people who turned eighteen years of age to sign a non-disclosure agreement stating they would not pass on the donor's details to their other siblings or post the details on social media. (This will only happen if you undergo fertility treatment overseas, but it still may impact your child's international siblings.)

Anonymity

While I believe anonymity will one day be banned because it's no longer a viable concept, there are many countries around the world that still provide this option and some that offer it as the only option. Please consider the long-term impacts for your child when you select an anonymous donor. Everyone has the right to know their genetic origins. The pain and trauma experienced by those who are unable to learn this information can be harrowing.

Questionable practices by international banks and agencies

> *My daughter had a brain lesion found at age seven. The* [US] *sperm bank's response* [was]*: 'Unless she's dying, we will not ask the donor any questions.'*
>
> **American recipient parent**

> ***Note:*** The US sperm bank referred to in the quote above is used by multiple Australian clinics.

It may interest you to know that, in cases where international banks and agencies are concerned, donors, recipient parents and donor-conceived people have reported many instances of questionable and unethical behaviour. Following are some of the recorded examples.

- Allowing sperm donors to donate for many years and, on some occasions, for more than two decades.
- Adding donors to their public website as 'new donor' when they have already created multiple children.
- Including false attributes in donors' profiles (for example, details of false careers and job titles).
- Digitally altering donors' photographs to make them appear more attractive.
- Editing donors' audio files to remove 'negative' comments.

- Using a different donor from the one a recipient parent selected.
- Inadequate medical screening of donors, resulting in inherited diseases.
- Continuing to use a donor when a genetic disease or abnormality has been identified.
- Refusing to update a donor's profile when that donor has been identified as a carrier of a disease.
- Failing to notify the donor and/or recipient parents, about a potential genetic disease or abnormality.
- Increasing the donor's worldwide family limit after children have already been born.
- Changing a donor's status from ID Release to anonymous after sperm has been purchased, despite other donor-conceived children already being born to that donor.
- Refusing to disclose to recipient parents exactly how many children a donor has created.
- Being unclear with donors about the number of children created from their gametes.
- Advising recipient parents who have requested information be exchanged with their donor (and vice versa), that it has been, when it hasn't.
- Not facilitating a request for contact when both the donor and the recipient parent have expressed a mutual desire to connect.
- Advising recipient parents that their donor cannot be located when, in fact, the donor has been providing updated contact information for years.
- Discontinuing the services of therapists whose role it is to screen potential donors if the therapists refuse to approve people who present with indicators of a personality disorder.

9

Choosing Your Donor[s]

My clinic told me not to think too hard about selecting a donor off their list, but I felt that wasn't great advice. I was prepared to wait and took ages to go through the list as more and more donors were added over several months. As soon as the right one appeared, I knew in my gut straight away and I'm really happy with my decision.

Australian recipient parent

The concept of choosing a person (or people) to be the biological parent(s) of your child is somewhat preternatural and generally evokes a reaction of curiosity and mild levity from most people. One-liners about 'dating sites', 'hot celebrity look-alikes' or 'good breeding stock' abound. People relate stories about choosing the tallest donor; the donor who's already got some good-looking or intelligent children out there; or writing donor names on pieces of paper, scrunching them up, throwing them on the floor and letting the dog choose—yes, really. While a bit of light-hearted banter is always good for the soul, what we also know is that comments of this kind are often considered offensive by donor-conceived adults. Indeed, the mere concept of choosing a donor from a catalogue is often triggering for them and, for some donor-conceived people, equates to a human shopping event.

So, what takes priority when choosing a donor? Some donor-conceived people consider personality to be more important than looks and it will mean children are more likely to be compatible socially and intellectually with their raising parents. Others feel that looks are important but should never be used to disguise the fact that a child is donor-conceived. Many feel health history is the most important factor and, while some donor-conceived people have little or no interest in their biological parent, some express that all they really wanted was someone who was willing to connect with them.

When it comes to selecting a donor, the decisions can be difficult and the choices limited. In all scenarios, the most important question to ask yourself is, 'How is my choice of donor(s) going to impact the one person who doesn't have a say in the decision-making process; the person who, at some stage in their life, may need information to help them form their sense of identity in the world; who may wish to locate and communicate with their biological parent (where they are not already known) and, possibly, have an ongoing relationship with them—as well as with the rest of their genetic family members.'

The reality is that at some stage in your child's life, the issue of a donor is no longer *your* story, but that of your child and, eventually, of your child's children as well. Choosing a donor is a decision worth taking a lot of time over. Think carefully about advice from well-meaning people who use statements such as, 'Don't overthink it.' If you are partnered, it's vital you make the decision together. Giving the partner who will be the child's non-biological parent the lead in the selection process may also assist them with ownership over the decision and help them with parent–child bonding.[79]

On the following pages, we will take a look at some of the things you might factor in when making your decision.

Medical history and screening

> *My donor has breast cancer run in his family. His grandmother died of breast cancer and his sister has breast cancer right now . . . makes me so nervous and upset. I emailed him asking him about the health history and he said everything was good and he's healthy. Come to find out by his cousin, she told us about the breast cancer. . . I'm pretty annoyed that he felt the need to keep that from us.*
>
> **American donor-conceived adult**

One of the eligibility criteria for donors is that they need to be healthy; this seems like an obvious standard. Donor applicants are required to provide an outline of their family's medical history, which generally includes information about siblings, parents, aunties, uncles and grandparents. For instance, is there a heart disease or breast cancer theme? Is there evidence of inherited diseases, such as cystic fibrosis or Huntington's disease, or another genetic syndrome? Some diseases will eliminate potential donors from the selection process, but only if those diseases are screened for.

While this might appear to be a fabulously safe and secure process, it is perhaps alarming to note that, for reasons of privacy, donors cannot usually be made to provide actual medical evidence of their family's good health and a rather large proportion of data is self-reported—in other words, there is an element of trust involved. It's also important to consider that, when the medical assessment is undertaken, it represents but a moment in time. For instance, if the donor is a young person, they may not have knowledge of any genetic issues in the family—some very old death certificates might only display, 'Died of old age'; and an inherited disease or disorder may not yet have presented itself.

Occasionally, there are reports of donors who discover an inherited disease at a later date and go to great lengths to locate the recipients themselves when they have had extreme difficulty convincing the international sperm or egg bank to pass on the information to recipient families. There are also reports of donors who have admitted to stretching the truth, particularly when they have received a financial incentive for their donation. Some donors might simply hide the truth about their health status,[80] while others might not even think to pass the information on.

Donor-conceived and adopted people are not usually considered eligible for gamete donation unless they have access to their biological family's medical history. But what if the potential donor is unaware of the circumstances of their own conception story—a scenario that applies to literally thousands of donor-conceived people. In situations such as this, donors may innocently self-report on their non-biological parent's medical information, all of which is useless for determining inherited risk. The result is that the risk of passing on unwanted (and unknown) genetic traits escalates, especially in the case of popular donors.

International donors

If you are selecting an international donor, there is a risk that the donor may not be screened effectively. Do you know what the screening process involves in your chosen country? Are all the tests displayed on the website actually being completed as claimed? You don't need to dig too deeply on the internet to find a multitude of lawsuits against US sperm banks, all of which bring to light some serious concerns about the donor screening process.

Known donors

If you are selecting a known sperm donor, to avoid the issues discussed above regarding 'Medical history and screening', the donor can attend a clinic or other screening centre to provide a sperm sample and complete the clinic's requisite testing process. Are you aware of your donor's medical history? Are you aware of their *family's* medical history? Is there a history of diabetes, high blood pressure, cancer or hip dysplasia? What are you and your donor's blood types? Do you or your donor have the Rh factor (previously called the Rhesus factor), a blood classification that can have serious implications for your newborn child?[81]

If you are using a known egg donor, the donor will be required to present their medical history to the clinic. In all cases, the potential risks inherent in self-reporting still apply.

When completing your research and narrowing down the donor selection process, a good question to ask yourself is: 'How might my child's health be affected if I select this donor?'

Genetic carrier screening

> *I made the decision to get tested for the maximum number of conditions after learning my little sister was affected by a rare genetic condition last year. We'd found a donor who was perfect and had already had genetic screening done. He was a carrier for spinal muscular atrophy (SMA), the leading*

> *genetic cause of infant death. My results came back and I was also an SMA carrier. It was disappointing to find out we could not use the donor, but were relieved we'd decided to get tested.*
>
> **New Zealand recipient parent**

If you or your donor are a carrier of a hereditary disease, or if you just want to check that you're not, it is possible to undergo genetic screening—in some clinics, it may be compulsory. There are many different testing options available and some will test multiple conditions (even numbering in the hundreds), including cystic fibrosis, spinal muscular atrophy and Tay-Sachs disease. Some inherited diseases can affect people with certain ancestral backgrounds at a higher rate than they affect others so, depending on the donor you choose, it is important to educate yourself on any known diseases, some of which can result in severe outcomes—including the premature death of children.

Your donor may have already undergone genetic carrier screening and, once tested, you can identify the risk of conceiving a child together. If your donor has not been screened but you have already undergone screening and have been shown not to be a carrier of any conditions, then the risk may be reduced. If your own results have indicated a risk, this may reduce your donor options.

If your chosen donor has not been screened, you can usually arrange for them to be tested—at your expense. Check with your clinic regarding screening options, or you can arrange for screening via your GP.

Epigenetics

Epigenetics is a field of science that studies how behaviours and the environment can impact the way genes work. Epigenetic changes refer to modifications to the DNA which determine whether genes are turned on or off, without actually changing the underlying DNA sequence or 'blueprint' of a person.

Epigenetics begin in the womb and regardless of whether the gestational parent is using donated gametes/embryos or their own, the gestational parent will still influence the activity of the child's genes—this includes factors such as diet, alcohol, stress levels, air quality, exposure to trauma, and so on. For example, measles contracted by a gestational parent can cause deafness in the child, lack of folate can cause issues with spinal development, and excessive consumption of alcohol can cause foetal alcohol syndrome. After a person is born, environmental influences continue to impact gene expression but, again, the inherited blueprint from each of the biological parents remains unchanged.

One of the questions that arises frequently on donor forums is whether a gestational parent using donated eggs can pass their DNA onto a child. The answer is 'No', they cannot. The gestational parent's genes will not show up on their donor-conceived child's DNA test.[82] Please be aware that some international websites grossly overstate the effects of epigenetics with claims like, 'If you use an egg donor, your child will absorb your looks, eye colour and beauty through the placenta!' This is not correct.

On the other hand, can the gestational parent influence the genes that are *expressed*? Yes, they can, and this influence continues throughout a child's life through nurture and environmental factors.[83] In other words, environment and genetics *both* matter.

Professor Tim Jenkins, a researcher in the field of epigenetics, has stated that 'who we are' is derived from multiple sources and it is empowering to know where we get things from—and it's not a one-way street; our children influence us as well! For example, the shape and size of a child's nose might be inherited from the donor, but the way in which they smile can come from their non-biological parent.

It's important to celebrate both.[84]

How much donor information do you want?

Australian clinic-recruited donors

If you are considering an Australian clinic-recruited donor, you will receive non-identifying information including some, or all, of the following details: date of birth, their age when they donated, hair and eye colour, build and weight, height, marital status, occupation, religion, country of birth, ancestry, highest education level attained, interests, personal and family health history, blood group, their reason for donating, current donor recipient pregnancies and any existing children (including the donor's own family *as well as* other donor-conceived children). Depending on the clinic, your donor may also have been provided with the opportunity to record personal information, such as their favourite colour and food, hobbies, likes and dislikes, a personal message for the future child about why they donated, and so on. The clinic may also provide a childhood photo of the donor.

International donors

Sperm donors

The amount of information provided about donors can vary between countries, but given the commercial nature of international sperm banks, they tend to provide very extensive donor profiles. They generally include all of the information as described for Australian clinic-recruited donors, *as well as* other information, such as audio files, emotional intelligence assessments, handwritten letters for the future children, childhood photos and, in some cases, adult photos.

Egg donors

In a similar manner to sperm donors, the amount of donor information provided about egg donors can vary significantly between countries. For instance, some egg agencies will provide vast amounts of information, including a comprehensive list of physical features and lifestyle habits and, in some instances, a short descriptive letter from the donor about their personality, likes and dislikes, education, life goals, and so on. Agencies might also list the locations to which donors are prepared to travel and whether costs will be covered or not. Depending on the country, donors may place stipulations on recipients to whom they *do not* wish to donate (for example, same-sex couples or single parents).

Alternatively, particularly in countries where anonymity is the only option, limited information about the donor will be available. This might include physical characteristics and age and may extend to personal details, such as hobbies, personality traits and the donor's reason for donating.

Embryo donors

Again, the amount of information you receive about your potential embryo donors varies significantly depending on the country where you source your embryos and the manner in which the embryos were created. For instance, if you travel to another country where *all* donors are anonymous, you will generally receive limited, basic information about the embryo donors, such as hair and eye colour, height, and so on.

Known donors

Sperm and egg donor

If you are using a known donor who you meet in person, you will see firsthand all of their physical characteristics such as height, weight, eye colour, hair colour and so on. You will hear them speak, you will be able to ask them why they wish to be a donor and what level of education they've achieved—and you will also be able to make a personal assessment of their character.

So how much donor information is enough for you? Donor-conceived people tell us the more information they have, the easier it is to build their sense of personal identity (see Chapter 14, 'Talking about Donor Conception'). So, if you're using a clinic-recruited or international donor, it's a good idea to purchase everything that's on offer: the audio file; the extra photos; the personal essay. It may cost you a bit more, but your child will probably thank you for it.

Despite this, it's important to understand that having a photo of your donor, a few measurements and a personal essay is no guarantee that your donor-conceived child will not experience challenging emotions about their conception story at some point in their lifetime.

Is your 'local' donor an Australian (or are they American, English, etc?)

> *One of the few things I'm grateful for in all of this is that my bio father is local.*
>
> **Australian donor-conceived adult (WA)**

Just because you select a donor through an Australian clinic's donor program, that doesn't mean the donor is Australian. While some clinics and public donor banks may require donors to be Australian citizens, most don't. As long as a donor has a temporary residence visa (or even a working holiday visa), a permanent address and three forms of identification, they can start donating—provided they also meet all of the other requisite criteria.

If this is an issue for you, ask the clinic about your donor's residency status prior to making your final selection and decide whether you are open to the risk of your donor decamping back to their country of origin (or elsewhere). Of course, even if your donor is an Australian citizen, it does not mean they may not, one day, choose to live overseas.

Likewise, if you choose an international sperm or egg donor, it is also possible they may not be a citizen or resident of that country. Some sperm and egg banks import gametes from other countries to include in their donor pool. Again, if this is an issue for you, check with your clinic and egg bank to confirm the donor's residency status.

Distance, language and culture

> *One of the issues parents really need to consider is the origins of their kids and what that actually means for the kid long-term. I mean, did you source a Ukrainian egg donor via the UK and a Spanish sperm donor from Denmark . . . while you live in Australia? And if you used embryo donors, how many times was your kid a leftover embryo that basically got 'moved on' multiple times? How will your kid find their bio-parents? How will they communicate when they might*

not even speak English? Will they have full siblings from the people who donated the embryo—who themselves may have used donor sperm and eggs—and then a handful of half siblings from the original egg donor and more half siblings from the original sperm donor? Please, please consider what this means for your kid.

Australian recipient parent

We know that donor-conceived people often wish to connect with siblings and their biological parents. If you select a donor on the other side of the country or the globe, consider that this will not make it easy for your child to connect. Furthermore, if you select a donor from a country with a primary language that is not your first language, how will your child manage the language and cultural barriers with their biological parent? It's also important to know that in some countries or among some religious groups, the donation of gametes and embryos is considered unacceptable. This could impact your donor's desire or ability to connect with your child because, in doing so, they may be risking personal shame and the censure of their family and community if their secret is discovered.

There are special groups within donor-conceived support groups for those struggling with cross cultural connections. It poses significant challenges. Apart from the obvious language and culture differences, economic considerations and time differences compound those difficulties.

Australian donor-conceived adult (NSW)

Yes, there are many incredible communication options these days, but most donor-conceived people say that talking to someone on Skype is not the same as meeting them and spending time with them in person. Distance makes it difficult to establish relationships.

So, while you may think that using an international donor is the best option for you right now, or perhaps it appears to be the *only* option, it's important to consider how that decision will impact your child's sibling and donor relationships long-term.

Physical features, race, ethnicity and the impact on your child

> *I don't look very much like either of my raising parents. There were small things—like I always hated my short, stubby fingers while my mum has gorgeous long elegant fingers. My great-grandmother on the donor's side published a few autobiographical books and mum read them. She called me one day in delight to tell me that my great-grandmother also complained about her short, stubby fingers! I didn't realise how much I'd always felt like I didn't belong until I had that moment of belonging.*
>
> **Australian donor-conceived adult (NSW)**

> *I don't mind being a different ethnicity than my parents who raised me. What I wish is that I had access to information and was able to celebrate that heritage as I was growing up.*
>
> **American donor-conceived adult**

The question, 'Should I choose a donor who looks like me?' is one that intended parents contemplate at length, some going to extraordinary measures to find the right 'match'. Is it actually important to you—and will it be important to your child?

What are the aspects you need to consider? Some of them are discussed on the following pages.

What is identity?

Before examining these questions, it's important to understand the concept of identity. Identity is a complex, enduring process that enables us to define 'who we are'. Identity refers to both the unique characteristics a person is assigned at birth (such as physical features, attributes and abilities) as well as personal identity which is shaped by cultural and social context through family, community, peers, other people and life experience.[85]

So, what happens when part of a person's identity is hidden or unavailable? Some donor-conceived people express anger if this information has been hidden deliberately in an attempt to cover up the fact they are donor-conceived. Others feel sadness that they are unable to complete the picture regarding the unknown parts of themselves; others are satisfied with simply having the donor's profile information. Some share a sense of confusion and loneliness because they look nothing like their family members. Regardless, it's impossible to know how your child will be affected and this is not something within your control. The effect on your child may not even become evident until adulthood, so it's important to be prepared for the full range of possible emotions whenever they may arise.

What is genetic mirroring?

> *Setting aside the obvious need for complete and current family medical history, there is also the matter of genetic mirroring and genuine curiosity. It is natural to wonder where specific traits, physical features, and attributes come from, especially when those pieces of our identity are not reflected in our social family.*
>
> **Tiffany Gardner (American donor-conceived adult)**[86]

Genetic mirroring is commonly described as being able to see yourself in the family around you. It contributes to identity formation, beginning the moment you are born. Newborns will search around and look for their gestational parent's face first. This then extends to other parents (if there is more than one), extended family, friends, and so on. The child will then learn to talk by watching and mimicking their parent(s); they will learn to read the subtle nuances of body language and facial expressions through those displayed by their parent(s); and will know the curves and contours of their parent's face intimately. So, later, when the child looks in the mirror, they seek to find the same shapes and contours in their own face. 'Oh! I've got this parent's nose . . . that grandparent's eyebrows . . .' The people around them will actively be looking for these resemblances and will tell them they see them as well. Of course, not everyone looks like their parents or their siblings, but children and adults alike will still express curiosity and speculation: 'I wonder where I got my pointy chin from; perhaps it was from a great-grandparent?' Why? Because it's instinctive—it makes a person feel safe and comfortable and these similar characteristics form part of a person's identity.[87] And genetic mirroring extends beyond appearance. It may not even be obvious. For example, a person may wonder why they are skilled at art, or why they're attracted to certain types of music, book genres or food.

> *I wish I could have a beer with him and look into the eyes of half of me.*
>
> **American donor-conceived adult**

But what happens when genetic mirroring is lost? What do children see in the mirror when they look nothing like their parents, or when one biological parent (or both in the case of embryo and double donation) is absent and no donor pictures are available? An American donor-conceived person shares their experience:

> *When I discovered the identity of the gamete donor my parents used to conceive me, it's made a lot more sense. Just knowing who my biological father is and his personality traits filled out a part of me missing for a long time. It is a lonely and confusing feeling not to look like the other people in your family.*

An Australian donor-conceived person shares an alternative perspective:

> *Ethnically and physically, my bio father and my Dad are similar enough that it's not obvious I'm not biologically related to Dad. But I still felt a keen desire to know the face of my bio father. It might raise less questions if you look like the donor you choose, but I suspect it's somewhat irrelevant to the donor-conceived person; looking like your family doesn't make you more of a family than someone who doesn't look like their family.*

For double donor-conceived and embryo donor-conceived, or where an anonymous donor has been used, the first time a person might experience genetic mirroring is when they meet a sibling or when they have their own children.

Choosing a donor of a different race

> *My donor was Cuban, and I was raised in a completely white washed, ultra conservative Christian household. I feel that my Cuban heritage was stolen from me, and it's one of the things that upsets me most. As a kid, I was naturally drawn to Hispanic cultures, and even started teaching myself Spanish when I was twelve. Now that I know (I found out that I was donor-conceived at age 37), I am learning and incorporating Cuban culture into my kid's lives as much as I can.*
>
> **American donor-conceived adult**

For many people, finding a donor with the same race or ethnicity as themselves is extremely important, but what if there is no one available? And what about *choosing* a donor of a different race or ethnicity? Much research has been done about transracial adoptees (when a child who is of one race or ethnic group is placed with adoptive parents of another race or ethnic group). So, what of your donor-conceived child? Research involving donor-conceived adults whose appearance did not match their parent(s) showed that many adults expressed discomfort regarding their differences and the experience of being constantly questioned.[88]

> *It has been a unique, challenging, and oftentimes lonely experience to be a donor-conceived person of color (Mexican American) adult and to grow up being raised by white parents in a predominantly white community. My moms are the best parents I could ever ask for, but they did not do ample if any research or preparation for this, i.e. raising a brown child as white parents, let alone a donor-conceived person of color. Please, please learn and read everything*

> *you can about how to be an Anti-racist white person/ white accomplice, and read everything you can about being a white mom raising a brown child and how to do this in a way that honors your child's roots from all sides of their heritage. Get your child connected to their Latinx community, things related to their culture, and build deep relationships with other Latinx people. Find good resources so they can all feel affirmed and nurtured in all their intersecting identities and lived experiences that may be different than your own.*
>
> **American donor-conceived adult of colour**

There are many factors to consider.[89] If you intend to be the parent of a transracial donor-conceived child, have you educated yourself on the meaning and effect of white privilege (if relevant to your situation)? Are you willing to accept your child's racial identity and discuss it openly with them? Are you prepared to have conversations about racism—and help your child develop coping strategies—particularly if you have never experienced racism yourself? Are you able to support your child when they are asked questions about whether they belong to your family? Do you feel equipped to teach your child about their ethnicity and cultural background when you are not part of that same ethnic group? Are you open to the possibility of creating a 'bicultural home' in which relevant art, crafts and books are displayed; and where food eaten and music played reflect your child's culture? Do you know where you might find people of the same race and culture with whom they can interact, or where you might source a suitable mentor or respected Elder? As a family, would you be open to learning a new language together?

What about health issues? Different races and ethnicities can be predisposed to certain inherited diseases and disorders. Are you aware of what these might be and how they could impact your child—and your child's children (and future generations)? For instance, will your local health professional and health system have expertise in the relevant condition? Will your child have ready access to emergency medical care for procedures such as bone marrow matches? Some races and ethnicities are more predisposed to conditions (including cardiovascular disease[90] and breast cancer[91]) that are not immediately life-threatening in childhood, but have a greater risk of presenting later in life. Will your donor-conceived child be made aware of these risks so they can take preventative measures? When they attempt to conceive their own children, will they be aware that those children could be at a greater risk of being carriers for disorders such as alpha thalassaemia or sickle cell anaemia, which can both lead to severe illness or early death?[92]

What about the everyday needs of your transracial child? Will they have access to appropriate hair and skin care? Will clothes shopping be challenging due to locally produced items not fitting their body shape and will they experience body dysmorphia as a result?

These are just some of the challenges a transracial child may encounter in their day-to-day life—and the challenges will not end in infancy or adolescence. You may be required to undergo extensive amounts of research. Do you feel able to support your child in these matters or know where to access appropriate support?

What's the answer?

What then, is the answer to the question of donor resemblance? I think it's fair to say the answer is not cut and dried, with a wide range of complex variables needing to be considered. There are certainly varied (and opposing) views on the matter.

From a practical perspective, the availability of clinic-recruited donors of a specific race or ethnicity is often limited, so more time may be required to find one. Alternatively, you might wish to reach out to everyone you know, including relevant racial or ethnic groups and, for First Nations people, suitable communities, asking for suggestions about people who may be willing to become a known donor.

In the end, perhaps the answer to this complicated question comes down to intent? For instance, are you intending to match a donor with your appearance so that you can keep your child's conception a secret—or is it, preferably, to ensure that donor conception is not always the main topic of conversation?

Perhaps the two most important questions to consider are: How might your decision impact your child's life, and are you in a position to support your child?

Prejudice within family constructs

Regardless of the type of donor you select, can you be certain they will be open to connecting with your child when your family is comprised of two mothers, or a transgender parent and a non-binary parent, or just one parent? If you are using a known donor selected from a matching site, have you discussed your family structure with that donor to ensure they are not homophobic or transphobic, or do not have a strong heteronormative stance towards family structures. This *could* be the difference between your child (should they wish to connect at a later date) being welcomed or rejected by their biological parent and their extended family.

Lifestyle preferences

If you are using a clinic-recruited or international donor, information about their lifestyle preferences (in varying degrees of detail) will be listed on their profile. Of course, this will not represent a complete picture of who they are. Some of it may not even be true, but at least it gives you an insight into the type of person your donor might be.

Many donor-conceived adults describe their biological parent as being very different from the profile their parents were given. For instance, is your donor religious? Are you? How do you feel about your donor having many gods, if you worship only one (or none)? Does your donor hold views at the other end of the political spectrum from your own? Are you a vegan activist while your donor is preparing their shotgun for duck season?

None of these things might feel important to you right now, but could they be important to your child later? Alternatively, does it matter (or might it even be important) that your child is exposed to alternative viewpoints?

Known donors

If you are using a known donor, you have the opportunity to dig deeper into their lifestyle preferences through preconception meetups and conversations. If you are not co-parenting, would you be comfortable with your child (and yourself) spending time in the company of this person?

If you intend to co-parent, have you considered what style of parenting appeals to you? You may have strong ideas based on the way you were parented, or perhaps you've observed your family and friends with their children and have a good sense of basic parenting principles that resonate for you.

What about your donor? Do you know how they and their partner might conduct themselves as parents, or significant influencers? More importantly, will your parenting styles be harmonious? People can have very different attitudes towards fundamental behaviours. Exposing your child to drastically different ways of living over alternate weeks may cause confusion and anxiety for all parties, especially your child. If the donor and their partner are going to play a parenting role in your child's life, make sure you all agree on the kind of lifestyle choices you desire for your child.

If you are a first-time parent, your attitudes and beliefs may change as you experience the realities of parenting, so it is probably a good idea to re-evaluate your situation at regular intervals. All of your co-parenting arrangements and shared parental responsibilities should be outlined in the legal documentation your lawyer drafts. (For more information about co-parenting see Chapter 6, 'Known Donors'.)

Donor age and related issues

How do you feel about your donor's age? Whether you consider them to be particularly young or, alternatively, on the aging side, there are some potential issues you may want to consider.

Younger donors

> *There are very predatory practices by fertility clinics, at least in the US, offering a lot of money to very young people in exchange for their gametes. Personally I don't think gamete 'donation' should be legal until twenty-five, the age when most people have a fully-functioning prefrontal cortex.*
>
> **American donor-conceived adult**

In Australia, clinics tend to advertise their egg donors as between twenty-one and thirty-six years of age (give or take a few years, depending on the clinic or public egg bank concerned). Most clinics also recommend that egg donors have completed their own families prior to donating, due to any associated risks which could affect their own ability to conceive (see Chapter 13, 'Being a Donor and How it Works'). Young people may still be allowed to donate if they insist they do not wish to have their own children.

If you are selecting a sperm or egg donor from a country where donors are paid, in some cases those donors will be in their teens (of minimum age eighteen years) or in their early twenties and attending university, because this is where banks and agencies tend to do a lot of their recruiting. An Australian recipient parent describes her experience:

> *Although I wanted an egg donor that was fertile, I also wanted someone a bit more mature than 'the youngest woman available', which is what they offered me.*

While a younger person's gametes may be more energetic and prolific than those of an older person—have you considered whether a teenage or twenty-something donor is fully cognisant of their actions? The prefrontal cortex (the rational part of the brain) is not considered to be fully developed until the age of twenty-five. This means that, until then, donors are processing information using their amygdala (the brain's processing centre for emotions) rather than making decisions based on good judgment and an awareness of the long-term consequences of their actions. Do they understand, for instance, that they are likely to be the biological parent of multiple children—who will grow up, wish to make contact and even to have a relationship with them? Have the donors completed their own families (this should be made clear on the donor's profile)? Do they even understand how conceiving multiple donor-conceived children could impact their own family, or their own children later in life? Some countries do not provide counselling to discuss these considerations with donors. And is an eighteen-year-old responsible enough to self-report the medical history of their family accurately? Are they even going to *tell* their family they are donating gametes and, as a result, be informed about the heart disease on their maternal side, or the haemochromatosis on their paternal side? If your donor is being paid (or significantly reimbursed via regular instalments), is the lure of that pocket money (or the Caribbean holiday) enough to justify a few untruths about their mental health issues or their late grandfather's bowel cancer? In eighteen years' time, will your now older and wiser donor have any regrets? More importantly, will they accept or reject your child's request for contact?

If you are using a younger known donor, similar implications may still apply.

Older donors

Fertility declines with age for all genders. For women and people who produce eggs, fertility starts to decrease slowly in their early thirties, diminishes more rapidly at around the age of thirty-five and, by forty years of age, the chances of conceiving and giving birth are halved. The risk of miscarriage, gestational diabetes, the need for caesarean section and stillbirth are also greater.

On the other hand, the uterus generally remains quite functional in older people and this explains why many people in their mid-to-late forties have success with donor eggs. Diminishing egg quality is the reason the age limit for egg donors is capped much lower than for sperm donors.

Likewise, the age of men and people who produce sperm can have a significant impact on the ability to conceive and give birth. For instance, when a sperm donor is over forty-five years of age, it can take five times longer to conceive using their gametes than it does for a donor in their twenties—and the risk of miscarriage is doubled. Children with older biological parents are also at a slightly greater risk of autism, birth defects and chromosomal abnormalities—such as Down's syndrome.[93]

If you are using a donor from an international sperm bank, donor eligibility is generally capped at around the forty-year mark (or younger) and you will be provided with the donor's date of birth. Likewise, the eligibility of Australian clinic-recruited sperm donors is generally capped at forty to forty-five years and, in some cases, the age is older than for international donors, primarily because Australian donors do not get paid and their donation is, therefore, an altruistic act. The result is that many men who donate have already had a family.

If you are using a known egg or sperm donor via a clinic, there may be some flexibility regarding their age, as long as you can demonstrate that you understand and accept the possible risks.[94] If you choose an older sperm donor (yes, there are known sperm donors who are active in their seventies), you may also want to consider the possible age range of your child's siblings and whether the donor will still be alive when your child reaches their teens.

Intelligence

> *Being gifted is not easy. It's not having every door opened. It's not succeeding in everything you do. It's not a walk in the park. It's isolating. It's not fitting in with your peers. It's being different. It's not being understood. It's a path not many tread. To have to navigate alone, with no footsteps to follow is hard. It's lonely. It's unnavigated with many branches blocking your path. To have known my gifted father and brother would have paved my way. Would have left the footprints for my gifted child to follow.*
>
> **Kate Richards (Australian donor-conceived adult [Vic.])**

Intelligence, like most aspects of what makes a human being, is affected by both genetics and environmental influences. Research indicates that factors such as nutrition, parenting and education can also have a significant impact.[95]

Many international sperm and egg bank/agencies conduct intelligence tests as part of their donor recruitment criteria and, in some cases, charge intended parents a higher rate for a donor with, for example, a PhD. Of course, there are no guarantees your child will inherit said genes.

Some donor-conceived people place intelligence in the highly offensive 'designer baby' category but, whatever your opinion, does having a high IQ actually equate to happiness? According to some studies, gifted children require significant amounts of support to help them achieve success in life and are at a higher risk of experiencing mental health issues.[96] For instance, unrealistic expectations are often placed on gifted children because their maturity does not match their intellect; there is a tendency to strive for perfectionism which can subsequently lead to a sense of failure, the risk of social alienation, and more.

You may be seeking an intelligent donor to match your own intellect or, perhaps intellect is of little importance to you. Either way, if your child's intellectual capacity is notably higher than yours (and your partner's), will you be able to keep up with the conversation at the dinner table? Anecdotal evidence from many donor-conceived adults indicates they recognised early on that they were significantly more intelligent than their raising parents.

How many children do you want?

Same donor; or different donor?

You may be happy if you conceive just one child but it is definitely worth considering from the outset how many children you would like and whether your donor can accommodate this. For example: Is your egg donor prepared to go through further cycles if you have no embryos left? Are they nearing the end of their donating life? Have you reserved extra vials of sperm with the clinic? If necessary, is it possible for you to purchase leftover vials of sperm from other families who have used the same donor and have completed their families? Is your known donor aware of your desire to have more than one child? Will they be available to help you?

Of course, despite all of your preparations, being able to conceive with the same donor may be beyond your control, leaving you in the position of needing to select a different donor for each of your children. Alternatively, you may have a child from a previous relationship and now wish to have another child using a donor. While this divergence does not have to be a showstopper, it is important to consider how multiple donors might impact the relationship between your children. For example, will one child successfully connect with siblings and the donor, while the other doesn't? Will one child go to their biological parent's house every second weekend, while the other stays with you? Can you be certain that your own family (parents, siblings, nieces and nephews, etc.) will accept a donor-conceived child as part of their family?

Like all things in life, experiences vary significantly. An American donor-conceived adult describes her experience as positive:

> *I'm sperm-donor conceived and my older sister is biologically related to both of my parents, and I have never felt 'lesser than' because of it, I'm actually very close with her.*

A Western Australian donor-conceived adult describes a different experience:

> *I have two sisters that I was raised with that are biologically my mum and dad's. It breaks my heart. I constantly feel like I'm grieving. I feel like I have less entitlement to my father than my sisters. I am the black sheep. The odd one out. The rebellious one. The different one. I will never feel like I fit in. I will always feel like I'm on the outside.*

Of course, it's impossible to know the answer to the questions surrounding multiple donors, and children may be able to navigate their own journeys, together and separately, without any issues. Or it may create problems such as jealousy, resentment, an emotional disconnect in your children's relationships, or a sense of isolation from their non-biological family.

Whatever your decision, make sure you educate yourself about the possible challenges for your unique scenario and be prepared to support and guide your children through any issues they may face.

Family limits and siblings

> *I encourage recipients of gametes to think about what it might mean to discover your thirteenth half-sibling on a DNA site when you're both adults, as that happened to me yesterday and will likely happen to your children. Do I reach out? How do I approach this subject? Do they know that they were donor-conceived? Do they want to connect with us? The questions are endless. Even if you ultimately develop a fantastic relationship with them, it's quite a bit of mental and emotional processing every single time one turns up—especially so if you feel that it's your duty to share the truth even if it's uncomfortable.*
>
> **American donor-conceived adult**

Have you considered how you would feel about the existence of half-siblings for your child, how many there might be and where around the globe they may be located? Note that US sperm banks ship their sperm to multiple countries around the world. What will happen if you discover your child has thirty siblings? Two hundred? Will you find yourself outraged at your sperm bank/clinic/prolific known donor? Nervous about the psycho-social impacts your donor-conceived children may experience as they move into their teens, and become young adults attempting to establish their identities in the world?

Despite the NHMRC *Ethical Guidelines* indicating that Australian clinics may not enter into contractual arrangements with overseas providers who offer practices that are considered unethical,[97] depending on the type of donor you choose, you may have little, or no control, over the number of siblings your child ends up with.

In many cases, like my daughter Lola's,[98] you may never know the final number.

Australian family limits

Australian family limits are significantly lower than countries such as the USA. Check to see the limits required by your local jurisdiction.

The NHMRC *Ethical Guidelines* direct clinics to take 'reasonable steps' to ensure the number of families created from a single donor are minimised.[99] Reasonable steps might include, for example: ensuring that, if the limit is five families, when a fifth person is pregnant with the same donor's sperm no one else can use it until all of their frozen embryos have been used; the intended parent fails to conceive and decides to try with a different donor; or the intended parent gives up trying to conceive. The family limit rule does not apply when an *existing* family wishes to have more children with the same donor.

Choice of donors

Sperm donors: Australian clinic-recruited donors

Clinics are required to ask sperm donors whether they have already donated elsewhere—including known donations. Nevertheless, it is not impossible for an Australian donor to withhold this information and end up producing large numbers of children in multiple states and territories, or even within the same state (although this is perhaps, less likely than international donors who are paid). If, on the other hand, the donor themselves wishes to limit the number of families, they can indicate this on their consent form at the clinic.[100]

Sperm donors: International donors

> *We have to keep track of stock right down to the last nut and bolt at work. How is it that human lives on this scale don't need to be kept track of?*
>
> **Australian recipient parent**

With regard to ART, all countries differ in their rules and regulations—or lack thereof. Regardless of this, Australian clinics which have service agreements with international sperm and egg banks and egg agencies must ensure that the manner in which gametes are obtained is consistent with Australian legislation and guidelines.[101] But does this always happen?

> *We chose a US sperm donor through our Australian clinic. The sperm bank told our clinic that we would be the first to use him. When our clinic checked, he had actually reached his family limit in Tasmania, NSW and QLD. The sperm bank said the Australian clinic is supposed to tell them if a donor has reached their limits, but he was still on their website as being available for Australians. That was a year and a half ago and he's still there.*
>
> **Australian recipient parent**

International sperm banks advertise their own family limits and the number should conform to the relevant country's rules and regulations, if any exist. International sperm banks supplying Australian clinics are supposed to work within the confines of Australia's state and territory family limits as part of their service agreement.

However, many sperm banks have what is called a *worldwide* family limit. And this is where the waters get a little murky.

> *There can't be 'limits' until they have accurate recordkeeping, which no sperm bank has.*
>
> **Wendy Kramer (founder of the Donor Sibling Registry)**

Some countries manage the family limits well; some have legislation; some rectify their processes when they make a mistake—others, not so much. And mistakes in governance happen. For instance, in 2017 in the Netherlands—despite there being a limit of twenty-five offspring per donor—one man donated at eleven different clinics across the country and produced over one hundred offspring. The donor said he did this because it made him 'feel helpful'.[102]

When it comes to the USA, a country which many Australian clinics use, sperm banks are not always legally obligated to stay within their advertised worldwide family limits. Sometimes a sperm bank will set a worldwide family limit for a donor and then a different family limit within the US—with the same donor. Some sperm banks advise that there is no worldwide limit; they just follow the guidelines for each country with which they work—but how many children does that add up to exactly?

Adding to the disquietude, some sperm banks, rather than employ people to follow-up the users of their donor sperm, place all of the onus on intended parents to report births. Sadly, many people do not complete this step for a variety of reasons, including: the belief that 'it's not the sperm bank's business'; or they don't want the sperm bank to keep their personal details on file; or the mistaken belief that the clinic has reported it for them; or they simply forget. The downstream effect of this truancy is that the sperm bank continues to promote the donor, their sperm continues to circumnavigate the globe and, as you can imagine, the worldwide family total can quickly transcend the definition of 'large family' and become something more akin to 'modest-sized principality'.

Furthermore, sperm banks have no way of tracking the secondary market when surplus vials of sperm are gifted or on sold to other families. Sometimes gametes are sold to clinics in other countries where there are no records kept. In addition, there is no tracking of surplus frozen embryos that may be on-donated several years later and many embryo donation programs still operate under total anonymity.

Some sperm banks won't even let a parent register a child's birth if they've used a leftover embryo created with donor gametes, because the parent is not the original recipient of those gametes.

And let's not forget those people ordering sperm and having it delivered to their front door (because you can do that in the USA) where it has been reported that other recipients arrived on said doorstep to split the cost of the vial.

And the siblings keep coming.

Even more disturbing, some sperm banks refuse to disclose how many children a donor has conceived, which naturally begs the question, why not?

But wait, there's more . . . To further agitate the millpond, there have been instances evidencing that Australian clinics do not necessarily check whether an international donor has also been used at clinics in other Australian states. The result is that while the Australian clinic is seen to be adhering to the relevant state or territory limit, no one is controlling the *total* number of children the donor conceives on our golden soil.

Exclusive sperm donors

If you have a lot of cash and you don't want anyone else to share your donor, some international sperm banks offer what they call 'exclusive donors' or 'limited donors'. There are various definitions of 'exclusive'—make sure you read the fine print. For example, in the case of sperm donors, you may be required to purchase the donor's *entire* inventory of sperm, however large or small. Alternatively, you may be required to pay a much higher fee than usual to access an exclusive donor's sperm or pay a 'package' rate; in other cases, there may be an option where a reduced number of families worldwide are able to access the sperm.

Some Australian clinics also offer exclusive donors (in some states, this is mandatory when using international gametes). This effectively means the donor's sperm cannot be sold anywhere else worldwide and the family limits can be adhered to closely within the relevant Australian state or territory. The downside is that you may be required to secure as many as ten vials of sperm (and potentially re-mortgage your house).

However, due to the lack of regulation and national registers in the USA (and in many other countries) it is not impossible that your 'exclusive' donor has presented himself at other clinics across the country (or in other countries) and made deposits there. Some donors have admitted on social media forums to 'donating' at multiple sperm banks; and some families have discovered via direct-to-consumer DNA testing that their donor was actively donating at more than one sperm bank. This, of course, means that there may be additional undisclosed offspring from Donor #1234, who is in actual fact also Donor #4321. Furthermore, there are no guarantees your exclusive donor has not already been active as a known donor or that he might choose to do so at a later stage. This means the only way of knowing whether your 'exclusive' donor service was upheld is via DNA testing later.

Known donors

If you are using a known donor, there is no legislation that covers the scale of their donation activities and there is a large degree of self-regulation required on the donor's part. This introduces an inherent risk regarding your donor's attitude toward family limits and has implications for you and your donor-conceived child. It is also important to consider how many children you wish to conceive and whether the one donor can fulfil your expectations.

Following are some topics for discussion with your known donor about siblings.

- If you wish to have a second or third child using the same donor, is the donor open to that possibility? Will they be available? What if your donor meets a new partner? Will they continue to commit to further conception attempts with you? If you are using an egg donor, are they open to undergoing another treatment cycle, if required?
- Has your known donor previously donated at a fertility clinic (or clinics)?
- Do you know how many other donor-conceived children your known donor already has? Do they?
- Does your donor know how many children they *intend* to have? Is it a reasonable number? Can you be sure they are telling you the truth? The donor's own children will be your child's siblings.
- Has your donor offered to help you conceive when you know they have told a different recipient parent they have finished donating?
- How will you and your child contact other (including future) recipients and siblings? For instance, is the donor open to forming a private group on a social media platform?
- Has your donor provided gametes to people who don't wish to have contact with other families, or might they do so in the future? If so, how do you feel about your child not being able to contact those siblings?

- If there is a genetic health issue with your donor or one of the children conceived by that donor, how will this information be disseminated to the families? Do you trust your donor to do this?

Implications of high sibling numbers

> *Just another DC day; I think I spotted at least ten different people today whose faces I studied intently, because something about them seemed similar to my own features and I wondered if they might be my half siblings. So weird to think this might be the closest I get to meeting some of them. Exhausting.*
>
> **Australian donor-conceived adult (Vic.)**

While it might seem like a lot of jolly fun to have siblings in the triple figure range—I mean, there's the free accommodation around the world; vast quantities of birthday gifts; and an endless supply of League of Legends™ players if it's past some people's bedtime. But there are also multiple issues to consider.

And the people most affected by this scenario are the donor-conceived children; especially when they grow up to become adolescents and adults. Although the risk of sibling numbers spiralling out of control is higher for sperm donors, large family groups can still occur for egg donors.

It's also important to know that Australian clinics who use sperm banks with large family limits might not be up for big conversations about accountability. So, you may be provided with the numbers and you may be provided with the choice, but what you may not hear is the multitude of problems having one hundred siblings creates for your donor-conceived child.

So I will share some of those with you on the following pages.

Medical conditions

> *My body is attacking itself. All they can tell me at this point is it's autoimmune and they think it's genetic. I, along with other siblings, have many health issues from our parents'*

donor. Well, we are 'doctor-conceived' unethically, but this still applies. It sucks going through this, and it sucks that I don't have medical history. I also have a clotting disorder and a gene mutation that causes other health issues. I have a biological father that could share health history that may be important and help me and my other siblings, yet he refuses.

Jacoba Ballard
(American donor-conceived adult; *Our Father* documentary)[103]

As described earlier, your donor-conceived child is not entirely safe from risk when it comes to inheriting a genetic disease or disorder from the donor. Of course, there are no guarantees for any of us, regardless of the circumstances of our conception. But, when an inherited disease does present itself and there are extremely large numbers of children running around bearing 50% of the donor's genes, this represents a problem of sizeable proportions.

I've known my bio father for seven years now and in the first few years he'd mention there was relevant medical information I needed, but he'd tell me another day. At this point I've given up. It feels awful to know that someone has information that might impact my health, but he doesn't want to share it for whatever reason and there's nothing I can do about it.

Australian donor-conceived adult (NSW)

The problem is also amplified when people don't report the birth of their child to the clinic, thereby contributing to the ongoing availability of the donor's gametes (which can amount to a significant number of families when international donors are involved). Inherited disease can also be problematic for people who choose not to have any contact with (or knowledge of) other donor recipients and subsequently 'miss the memo' about commonalities that may point to potential issues with the donor. At this point you may be thinking that *surely* the bank will pass on any medical concerns to all of the other donor recipients so they can be aware of a potential issue. And yes, in many instances, they will—but, sadly, history tells us that some international banks can be averse to sharing this kind of information unless it can be proven the situation is 'life and death'.

If you use a known donor who has plans to populate the planet, similar issues apply. In this case, the risk of inherited disease is possibly even higher. For instance, has a known donor with this kind of grandiose ambition undergone screening procedures to detect inherited disease? Do all of the recipient parents from that donor keep in touch with each other? Do they even know about each other, particularly in cases where the donor has lied about his existing donor-conceived children? That particular scenario would require each recipient to inform the known donor of a successful live birth and the donor to subsequently inform each recipient—past, current and ongoing. Yes, it does happen via private social media groups for instance but, all too frequently, some families choose not to participate.

Consanguinity

> *I will never know all my siblings. Never. You just can't form meaningful relationships with that many people. I will never even know their names. If I have children I will need to warn them to be careful they don't shag their cousins. They would be likely to have 60+ in my state of Australia.*
>
> **Australian donor-conceived adult (WA)**

Consanguineous is a term from the Latin meaning, 'the condition of being blood relations'.[104] The possibility of people who are related forming a relationship or conceiving a child is a scenario that is frequently scoffed at, with the risk cited as highly improbable. But it does happen.[105] And is the possibility of consanguinity increased when extremely large numbers of siblings exist? What are the chances? Many donor-conceived people relate stories of discovering they lived next door or 'down the road' from a sibling, or went to the same school or college as them, or worked together. But what about the thousands of people who don't know they're donor-conceived?

Opinions and statistics notwithstanding, donor-conceived adults tell us the fear of consanguinity is real and takes a heavy psychological toll. If you choose a bank and you are not aware whether they will keep on selling your donor's gametes far and wide, could you be placing your donor-conceived child at risk of consanguinity? Alternatively, if you use a prolific known donor—a person on a mission to mark their territory and who may have limited their donations to a small region or district—could the risk be even greater?

Genetic sexual attraction

The term, 'genetic sexual attraction', refers to the attraction that arises towards siblings (and cousins and parents) who first meet or are reunited as adults. In circumstances where relatives grow up in the same residence, humans appear to have developed an inbuilt mechanism that takes effect at an early age and desensitises them from viewing each other as sexual prospects later. This is known as the 'Westermarck effect' after Finnish anthropologist, Edvard Westermarck.

There have been several studies related to Westermarck's theory (which some consider to be pseudo-science) and, while it is unclear whether other factors contribute to the lack of sexual attraction towards family members who grow up in the same household, there are people around the world (mothers and sons; daughters and fathers; half-brothers and sisters, etc.) who claim to have experienced genetic sexual attraction.[106]

With regard to gamete donation, the combination of vast numbers of children from a single donor (and the element of secrecy in many cases) means donor-conceived people are potentially at risk of genetic sexual attraction. And while the situation is somewhat disquieting, people suffering from the effect describe a genuine sense of powerlessness and a terrible internal struggle arising from loving a person that society says they must not.

Connecting with the donor

If you choose a donor who has children by the dozen (or the hundred), is that person going to want to connect with your child? While it is true that there *are* donors out there with very large numbers of children who are happy to connect with some or all of them, it seems likely that many (once they comprehend the sheer number of humans they've created) will make a hasty exit out the rear entrance when donor-conceived child 15 of 150's email arrives in their Inbox (see Chapter 15, 'Donor and Sibling Linking').

Searching for siblings

> *As one of a large donor sibling group I can promise you it's not all it's cracked up to be. In fact, every time I get another message from Ancestry or 23&Me I start to have an anxiety attack. So much pain and shared loss.*
>
> **Australian donor-conceived adult (NSW)**

When a person discovers they are one of many, a desire to find all of their hundred or so siblings can become an all-consuming life project—an obsession. While some people enjoy this super-sleuthing exercise, others arrive at a point they describe as fraught with anxiety, sadness and an overwhelming helplessness—especially when some of their siblings express shock, denial or disinterest in connecting. In some cases, a person might choose to sever a connection with newly discovered siblings, because the pain transference proves too unbearable.

Bearing the burden of decisions

For more information see Chapter 14, 'Talking about Donor Conception'.

Donors and sibling linking

For information on contact and connection with donors and siblings see Chapter 15, 'Donor and Sibling Linking'.

Signing an agreement

If you are using a clinic-recruited donor, the donor will sign documentation indicating they do not have an intention to claim parenting rights and, conversely, intended parents will sign documentation ruling out their intention to claim child support payments from the donor. International sperm and egg banks/agencies *usually* require you to sign documents with similar stipulations (see Chapter 8, 'Choosing an International Sperm/Egg Bank, or Egg Agency').

In the case of a known donor, it is absolutely vital to make agreements about a multitude of issues and a preconception agreement outlining your intentions and your roles is a very good idea (See Chapter 16, 'ART Regulations and Ethical Guidelines').

To pay or not to pay for a donor?

> *Having been born in the '70s when this procedure was provided free of charge to my parents, I'm so glad I wasn't paid for and picked out of a catalogue. I worry for donor-conceived people conceived in later years and how they will feel about their parents paying a lot of money for them and selecting desirable characteristics from a catalogue.*
>
> **Australian donor-conceived adult (Vic.)**

A friend of mine once told me that the state of her children's bedrooms was similar to a post-apocalyptic landscape, complete with rubble and toxic fumes. She simply couldn't get them to lift a finger (or a pair of smelly socks), so she started paying them. Not very much—just two dollars a week—but the kids quickly did the maths and whipped themselves into action. Every morning their beds were made, dirty clothes lifted from the floor, shoes lined up in the wardrobe. My friend was ecstatic—her house was clear; her mind open.

About two weeks in, she asked her ten-year-old daughter to feed the cat.

'I will if you pay me', she said.

While paying a child to feed the cat does not exactly have the same social, ethical and physical ramifications as paying a person to 'donate' their gametes, the issue of payment does raise some interesting questions. Certainly, when it comes to blood donations, the World Health Organisation recommends that the safest way to collect blood is from people who have volunteered because evidence suggests that, when payments are made, screening standards can be lowered, donors can be dishonest and companies can cut corners.[107]

But what about donor conception? In countries where donors are paid, could the pursuit of a cash reward foster unwanted behaviours; a few little half-truths; some outright lies? When responding to a question in the donor screening test about recreational drugs, might the potential donor answer 'Never', while reflecting on last weekend's rave party? What of the donor's family's medical history for the previous three generations? Did their father and grandfather really die of heart disease simply because they both consistently inhaled cigarette smoke for forty years, or is there something else more sinister at play in the donor's genetic makeup? Could the clinic or bank potentially overlook a minor discrepancy if they have donor recipients trampling the Odontoglossum orchids to get to their front door but not enough 'product'?

Another more practical issue to consider with payments to donors is how this could affect the relationship between the donor and their donor-conceived children. For example, when something is delivered with beneficence it generally creates a sense of connection between the giver and the receiver. On the other hand, a contractual obligation is usually concluded when payment is delivered. So does this mean there is a possibility a paid gamete provider may feel little or no sense of connection with their donor-conceived children?[108] If so, does this create the potential for an adverse outcome when your child attempts to connect with the donor in the future?

> *I'd feel uncomfortable telling a donor-conceived person that I donated because I wanted a car. It reduces the donation to a dollar value. I'd prefer them knowing it was altruistic and done purely to help.*
>
> **Australian egg donor**

It's also important to consider how your donor-conceived child-adult might feel about the fact that you handed over cash to create them. For instance, many donor-conceived people feel like a commodity and consider the monetary transaction and the corresponding marketing terminology to be repugnant.

Debate over the commercialisation of the donor industry continues. Nevertheless, given it is illegal to trade in gametes in Australia (see Chapter 16, 'ART Regulations and Ethical Guidelines'), people are generally donating for altruistic purposes.

Finances: Who pays?

When you choose a donor from a clinic's donor program or a sperm or egg bank, the future financial responsibility for the child is clearly defined—it is yours and yours alone.

If you are using a known donor and you are not intending to legally co-parent, then you should have full responsibility for all costs involved, including medical testing, ART treatment, and the costs of pregnancy, childbirth and parenting. If your donor has travel costs related to screening and conception arrangements, it is acceptable to reimburse them for reasonable out-of-pocket expenses, although legal advice should be obtained to ensure no breach of the law occurs. If your donor contributes financially to your ART treatment or in any other capacity throughout your child's life, this fact may be considered by the Family Court should a parenting conflict ever arise.

If you and your donor are co-parenting, an in-depth discussion and subsequent agreement about finances is vital. Topics for discussion might include the frequency of financial contributions, including payment for private health insurance, schooling, special events such as school camps and birthdays, and so on. It's also important to discuss financial and legal matters such as superannuation and wills—and whether your child might be named as a beneficiary. All of your co-parenting arrangements and shared parental responsibilities related to finances should be outlined in your legal documentation. (For more information about co-parenting see Chapter 6, 'Known Donors', and Chapter 16, 'ART Regulations and Ethical Guidelines'.)

Anonymity

For more information on anonymity see Chapter 16, 'ART Regulations and Ethical Guidelines'.

Embryo donation

The big difference with embryo donation is knowing it's random chance that put you where you were. That could become a big issue if the two families are hugely different in some way (wealth, parenting, etc.) as all children will be aware it was the luck of the draw. It would be equally devastating for you if your own children (that you're raising) wished they'd been the donated embryo because 'they get to go to Disneyland each year', for example. Of course, these things can always be navigated but it's well worth you both thinking about how you'll deal with that situation if it arises. How will you handle your own feelings enough to support your child if they're resentful of their entire lives coming down to luck? Many embryo adopted children may never have any negative feelings about it—but it's important to prepare for the possibility.

Australian donor-conceived adult (NSW)

While embryo donation may feel like a more appealing option, because you don't need to undergo a stimulation cycle, or select individual gametes—and it's cheaper—embryo donation deserves special consideration. Why? Because children conceived via embryo donation often have full siblings who are now separated or 'split' from each other, which opens up the potential for psycho-social issues. Concerns include the possibility of the child feeling they were 'the one that was given away' or abandoned by their biological parents, or that they were a 'leftover'.

On the flip side, how might the children who are living with their biological parents feel about having full siblings they don't get the chance to grow up with? As a result, many donor-conceived people are opposed to embryo donation, or believe that (like adoption) it should only ever be done as an open arrangement, involving the donating and receiving families establishing mutual trust *before* ART treatment takes place and continuing afterwards to ensure siblings and parents connect regularly. As an extension of this, many people also believe that embryo donation should only be conducted with one other family; in other words, an embryo is only passed on once.

For intended parents undergoing embryo donation, counselling sessions are required to cover the potential long-term psychological implications for an embryo donor-conceived individual whose embryo was passed on multiple times.[109]

Of course, your children may have no issues whatsoever about having resulted from embryo donation, but no one can know that ahead of time. Whatever your own feelings about embryo donation, make sure you do all the research you can; talk to adults who were born as a result of embryo donation, if possible (there are a few around); and be prepared to guide and support your child through any feelings and emotions that arise about their conception story.

10

Further Research Tips for Selecting Clinics, Countries and Donors

In addition to all of the questions you might ask your clinic, bank, agency or even your donor (if you're using a known donor), there are several other research methods that can take you 'direct-to-the-source'. Many online sites and social media forums exist on which people who have used the same clinic, sperm bank, egg agency, or even your donor, can offer firsthand experience. The information you uncover may enable you to make a more informed choice and, in some instances, could prevent a disaster.

It's important to remember that while, in some instances, the information could be crucial to your decision-making process, in other instances it may be just someone else's opinion. It's vital you maintain a clear vision of your personal needs, your standards and ethics and, most importantly, the needs of your donor-conceived child.

Social media and parenting websites

Social media is an excellent way to educate yourself about all things donor conception. On all platforms, sites abound for donor recipients, donors and donor-conceived people, as well as other impacted family members such as donors' partners and children. Independent Australian and international parenting websites provide the option of reading existing threads, asking questions and conversing with people who have information about the clinic, agency, bank or donor you are considering.

You will also find multiple social media groups specifically for Australians trying to conceive, as well as for families who already have donor-conceived children. Some donor matching sites also provide information and recommendations about people's experiences with Australian clinics and fertility specialists.

On these forums you can ask anything about: local clinics and specialists; Centrelink and Medicare payments; when to talk to your child about their conception story; local events at which people might physically meet up; and, of course, whether anyone has already used your donor.

International groups also exist in which recipient parents, donors and donor-conceived people offer advice and commentary on anything from: media articles; research papers; worldwide activist groups; advice for parenting donor-conceived children; DNA testing; and, again, whether anyone has used your sperm or egg bank/agency. It's useful to know that sometimes recipient parents find mixed groups (donors, recipients and donor-conceived people) confronting when some donor-conceived people express anger, grief or trauma about their conception story, or the problems they've experienced as a result. It's important to remember that your own child may experience similar emotions as they get older, and being prepared for such a response could help you to avoid similar scenarios as well as manage your own child's donor-conceived-related questions and issues. (See Chapter 14, 'Talking about Donor Conception'.)

In some instances, you might also find groups whose sole purpose is to provide a medium for impassioned recipient parents to share contemptible stories about specific organisations. These groups are very handy if you wish to uncover details relating to a bank's processes or communication policy (or lack thereof) and may even result in you selecting a different bank, and, subsequently, a different clinic—or even a different type of donor.

The online groups are usually private and require you to disclose some information about yourself prior to being accepted. Once you're on, it's a good idea to take some time to watch and wait, review the group rules, read some of the threads to identify the tone of the group and to check whether your questions have already been answered—then, go ahead and ask in an appropriate manner. You can communicate directly with the relevant people on the forums and make an informed decision about where, or where not, you wish to place your trust. In some cases, you may make lifelong friends.

Of course, let's not forget that social media is full of 'experts'. This means you need to use discernment and critical thinking when determining whether a person providing 'advice' is actually in a position to do so. Sometimes people can provide misleading or incorrect information; and some groups might feel toxic and harmful. Join multiple groups, ensuring at least some of them provide access to donor-conceived voices—and trust your gut when determining whether each group is right for you.

Donor and sibling linking sites

For more information on donor and sibling linking sites see Chapter 15, 'Donor and Sibling Linking'.

Lawsuits

Given the demand for fertility services and the related complexities involved, the fertility industry can be a highly litigious area. Use Google and social media groups to find out whether the clinic, sperm/egg bank or agency you are considering has a trail of litigation stories as long as the Hume Highway. Also look at the reasons why this is the case. Based on your findings, you may wish to find a new international sperm or egg bank and/or a new Australian clinic.

Sadly, overseas fertility companies having a long list of associated litigation stories does not seem to deter Australian clinics from doing business with them.

If you are using a known donor, you may also consider informing yourself about previous and existing legal cases involving parentage and parenting orders to ensure you fully understand the ramifications of using a known donor (see Chapter 16, 'ART Regulations and Ethical Guidelines').

Respect and understanding

While doing some research on your potential donor is a great idea—and you may receive friendly, welcoming responses from some recipients—it is important to note that some people find the concept offensive. For instance, imagine you come across a request on your social media feed that reads, 'Hi mamas! I'm thinking of using Donor B45 and am wondering if he makes pretty babies/big babies/intelligent babies/autistic babies', and so on. Or the person who requests photos of children so they can decide whether they like the look of what they see and, subsequently, which donor to choose. Would you respond to requests of this type, or would you scroll on down? And why might 'research' of this kind be deemed offensive?

Some donor recipients (and many donor-conceived people) find the notion of this type of research a bit too close to a shopping experience and a try-before-you-buy scenario. The commodification of children, or the 'designer baby' concept, is an idea that trails closely behind.

So, while it is a truly remarkable experience to connect with your child's siblings, if you intend to use these types of groups to reach out to existing donor recipients before selecting your donor, ensure you use language that shows respect, provide details about the reason for your search and be open to the possibility of silence in response.

Summary of Part 3: 'Making decisions'

> *Will your donor-conceived child be thanking you during their twenty-first birthday speech, or will they be saying, 'What the hell were you thinking?!'*
>
> **Kate Bourne (former Chair of the Australian and New Zealand Infertility Counsellors Association)**

One thing is certain: there are no guarantees in life. But if we can take measures to minimise the risks and conceive consciously then, surely we owe it to ourselves, our donor and, most importantly, our children to do so. In the end, only you can decide which donor is right for you (and from where you select that donor). And whether you like it or not, the answer you come up with will determine a lifelong connection (be it mental, emotional, spiritual, physical, genetic, or all of these) between you, your child, your child's children, your donor and your donor's family.

Should you resist the temptation to play down vitally important issues that arise because you feel grateful you have found a willing donor, or a clinic that offers you a great payment plan, or because you just feel desperate to get started? Do you feel as though you're in a position to make deliberate and considered decisions?

Whatever your situation, allow yourself plenty of time, sit in contemplation and ask yourself, 'is my decision centred on the best interests of my future child?'

Part Four: Assisted Reproductive Technology [ART], 'At-Home' Insemination and Conceiving Consciously

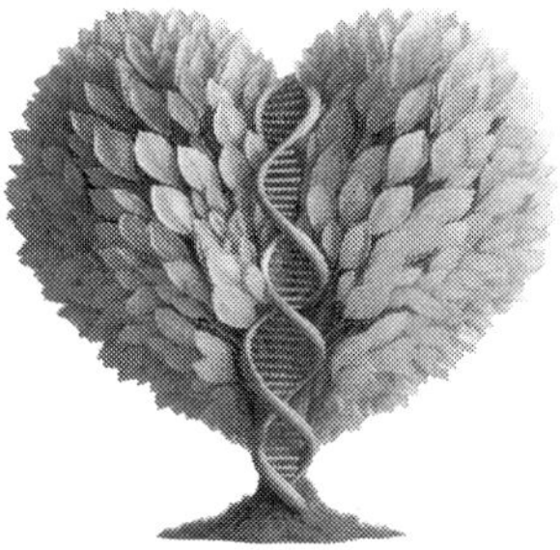

Nothing about this journey is simple is it? After multiple failed attempts at IUI with my known donor, one attempt at IVF, two with ICSI (and a couple of miscarriages), I've finally been blessed with my precious daughter. I also feel like I've got a degree in acronyms.

Australian recipient parent

What do IVF, ICSI, IUI and ICI stand for? What's a FET and do I have to do it? 'ART': isn't that a painting or a sculpture? Oh, so many acronyms! What do they all mean and how does it all work? Where does Medicare fit in? What are the costs involved?

The next two chapters tell you everything you need to know about the available methods of conceiving with a donor, as well as some important tips and suggestions for preparing your body for pregnancy and for determining whether your donor's lifestyle is compatible with your intention to conceive consciously.

If you're not quite ready to make decisions about conception options and preparing for pregnancy, skip this part and come back to it later.

11

Assisted Reproductive Technology [ART], 'At-home' Insemination, Success Rates and Costs

> *Based on my own experience and being steered in the wrong direction multiple times, my suggestion would be to investigate each of the options available to you using independent, scientific medical sources online. In other words, information NOT associated with a clinic. Have a consultation with your GP, do a full medical, Pap smear and breast examination, have a conversation about trying to conceive and then do a lot of your tests upfront because you might need to address these things before you try to conceive, e.g. iron, vitamin D, rubella antibodies, etc. Then ask your GP about all of the available options such as IUI, IVF, etc. so that you're armed with all of the information. Doing these things before you start might also save you lots of money, especially if you're using a clinic.*
>
> **Australian recipient parent**

Experimentation with sperm is not a new phenomenon and, prior to the twentieth century, was generally performed without consent. Other equally questionable practices surfaced over the ensuing years and it wasn't until 1953 that the first successful human pregnancy using artificial insemination was reported.[110]

Egg donation, on the other hand, is a significantly more complex process and did not enter the picture until the early 1980s. The first successful pregnancy using donated eggs occurred in Australia in 1983, although this did not result in a live birth.

Technology is constantly evolving and new techniques are being introduced all the time. With this in mind, how do you navigate the complex world of assisted reproductive technology (ART), or 'at-home' insemination if that is your preferred method?

What are the treatment options available?

What methods for achieving a pregnancy are available for people who need the assistance of a donor to build their family?

The following pages outline the steps involved, the potential risks and the people to whom the process is best suited. If you choose to undergo ART treatment at a clinic, it's important to be aware that not all options are available at all clinics. Ensure you check the available options before deciding to go ahead with a particular clinic, agency or donor.

Artificial Insemination (AI)

> ***Note:*** The use of donor eggs or embryos requires undergoing some form of ART treatment and cannot be achieved via artificial insemination.

The term artificial insemination (AI) refers to the process of inserting sperm into a person's reproductive tract with the aim of creating a pregnancy by means other than sexual intercourse. The intent of AI is to give the sperm a head start by placing them in the general vicinity of their end goal, although they still need to work to get there and fertilise the egg.

Insemination can be completed in different ways and the processes are named according to the location of the reproductive tract at which the semen is injected (for example, intravaginal and intrauterine).

How do intravaginal insemination (IVI) and intracervical insemination (ICI) work?

Intravaginal insemination (IVI) is the simplest of all insemination techniques and involves depositing semen via a syringe into the vagina during ovulation. Intracervical insemination (ICI) is similar to IVI in that it uses a syringe to place the semen but, with ICI, the semen is placed directly inside the cervix. In both cases, unwashed or raw semen is usually used, however frozen semen, once thawed, can also be used.

To successfully undergo ICI, you will need to understand the theory behind when people are most fertile and, more importantly, you will need to have a heightened awareness of your own menstrual cycle so you can identify when you are ovulating. You will also need to communicate clearly with your donor about the timing and check whether they are available on call and willing to refrain from sexual activity a few days prior to donating; enabling them to produce the peak number of motile sperm and potentially increase the likelihood of conception.

Artificial insemination can be performed during the course of a natural menstrual cycle or using hormones to artificially stimulate the ovaries.

There are many websites that provide detailed instructions on how to perform ICI effectively and a multitude of tools are available for purchase such as semen collection cups, syringes, conception kits, ovulation test strips and pregnancy tests.

Both IVI and ICI are suited to at-home insemination treatments for people who have no known fertility problems (such as endometriosis or blocked fallopian tubes) and are using a known donor with a good sperm count, a good sperm motility score (their forward progressive movement) and good sperm morphology (size, shape and appearance).

Benefits

Attempting ICI at home can offer several advantages. First, the process is free, aside from any medical testing you and your donor may undergo and, second, you can make several attempts at conception in the same monthly cycle.

While research indicates double insemination may increase the chance of pregnancy for heterosexual couples whose infertility is already known, the results are less clear for single women and lesbians using donor sperm.[111]

How does intrauterine insemination (IUI) work?

If you intend to carry out the insemination process at a clinic, intrauterine insemination (IUI) will be the technique offered. This is a more intricate procedure than IVI and ICI and requires medical training, so it is not usually carried out at home. The process of IUI involves using a speculum and a small flexible catheter to transfer specially washed semen directly into the uterus. The semen is either collected from the donor at the clinic immediately after masturbation or, in the case of a frozen sample, thawed and prepared. Chemicals called cryoprotectants are added to the frozen sperm to prevent damage caused by ice crystallisation. The preparation process involves analysing and washing the semen to remove any impurities, and any non-motile sperm or disease-carrying material—leaving only the motile sperm. While it's okay to insert unwashed sperm into a vagina, it can be dangerous to insert it directly into the uterine cavity because it *may* cause severe reactions such as nausea, vomiting, cramping and intense pain.

Intrauterine insemination can be completed using your natural cycle, or with the assistance of fertility medication to stimulate the release of multiple eggs. Completing IUI through a clinic normally involves tests such as blood monitoring of follicle development and ultrasounds. Unless you are using your own known donor, clinics do not generally allow multiple IUI attempts during one cycle due to the scarcity of clinic-recruited sperm donors and the small number of samples collected.

The IUI process is suited to people who have no known fertility problems and are using a donor with good-quality sperm. It is also suited to people who wish to minimise the health-related risks associated with IVF and, where frozen sperm is used, are not wanting to rely on the physical availability of their donor. Some research indicates that IUI is not very effective for people with endometriosis or people of 'advanced maternal age' (defined, sadly, as people over thirty-five).[112] As a result, many clinics rule out IUI for people above this age and may suggest the significantly more expensive IVF treatment as the next step.

Benefits

Undergoing IUI at a clinic means a specialist is able to assist you with tracking your cycle. The clinic's screening tests also mean a reduced risk of STIs and inherited diseases. Clinic-administered IUI also means your donor will be required to attend one or more counselling sessions. While this may seem disagreeable and time-consuming, it is essential that donors understand the long-term ramifications of what they are doing.

Using a clinic to undergo IUI with your known donor means you have the option of using frozen sperm. This means your donor need not concern themselves with sexual abstinence and other lifestyle choices, such as avoiding alcohol consumption prior to conception. You also don't need to be concerned about any sexual activity your donor may have between conception attempts; and you don't need to rely on their physical availability during your fertile window.

Risks of artificial insemination

Immediate risks following IVI, ICI and IUI include the possibility of infection after the treatment and vaginal bleeding if the syringe is not used correctly during ICI. While undergoing IUI at a clinic significantly reduces the risk of diseases transmitted via body fluids (including HIV and hepatitis), insemination at home without screening your donor places you at risk. Insemination at home removes the risks associated with direct sexual contact (such as herpes), but you could still be at risk of diseases transmitted via body fluids (including HIV and hepatitis), and your child could be at risk of genetic diseases (such as cystic fibrosis and Huntington's disease).

When undergoing IUI with a clinic-recruited donor or an international donor, the risks are not removed completely but they are greatly reduced because the sperm will undergo screening. However, the sperm will be frozen and thawed, a process that can cause significant damage to sperm cells and reduce the number of viable sperm available from the original sample.[113]

If you are using fertility medication together with IUI, there is a risk of developing ovarian hyperstimulation syndrome (OHSS), a dangerous and potentially life-threatening condition (see Chapter 13, 'Being a Donor and How it Works'). Clinics use blood testing and ultrasound to closely monitor patients for OHSS throughout the process of IUI.

The use of fertility medication can also raise the risk of multiple pregnancies due to more than one follicle maturing. Other side effects of using fertility medication can include drowsiness, depression, mood swings, weight gain, hot flushes, nausea, bloating, breast tenderness and vaginal irritation.

In vitro fertilisation (IVF) and Intra-Cytoplasmic Sperm Injection (ICSI)

The term 'in vitro' refers to a biological process that is performed in a culture dish or outside of a living organism. This means that in vitro fertilisation (or IVF) is the process of using sperm to fertilise an egg *outside* of the human body. Louise Brown (born in England in July, 1978) was the first baby conceived via IVF.

How do IVF and ICSI work?

In a typical monthly cycle, the body releases one egg. During the IVF process, hormone therapy involving multiple injections of varying medications aims to stimulate the development of multiple mature eggs—monitored with blood tests and intravaginal ultrasounds. This process of 'superovulation' is often referred to as a stimulation cycle, or 'stim cycle'. The growth of the follicle (where the eggs reside) is monitored closely, again via blood tests and ultrasound, to achieve the optimum number and size of follicles. Thirty-six hours prior to the egg retrieval process, hormone medication is self-administered via an injection, known as the 'trigger shot' or 'trigger injection'. This prompts the body to release the eggs at the right time.

Egg retrieval, also known as 'pick-up', is then undertaken when you are under general anaesthetic or light sedation. The process involves an ultrasound-guided needle which passes through the vaginal wall to reach the ovary and individual follicles. The needle is inserted into each follicle where a mature egg is then literally sucked out. The process is repeated for each follicle in both ovaries.[114] The eggs are then placed in a dish with sperm that have been collected, washed and prepared. The sperm are then left to locate and naturally fertilise the egg—hopefully!

The ICSI process differs in that, rather than using the 'may the best sperm win' approach, an embryologist carefully selects one individual sperm using a sophisticated microscope and injects it directly into the egg. Embryologists are required to undergo specialist training to perform the ICSI process and it takes many months to learn. The ICSI process was first developed for couples experiencing male factor infertility so, unless this describes your sperm donor, it may feel frustrating to hand over extra cash to your clinic. In fact, research conducted in 2018 indicated that ICSI resulted in a rate of live births similar to that of IVF where no male factor infertility existed.[115] Some of the reasons clinics use ICSI is because sperm may be in short supply or a donor does not have a high sperm count. Using ICSI means the sperm sample can be divided and used multiple times which, in turn, provides greater opportunities for conception—especially if you want siblings from the same donor. Another reason ICSI is used is to prevent more than one sperm penetrating the egg, thereby avoiding the chance of a multiple pregnancy.

If you don't care for your chosen clinic's rules about ICSI, you're entitled to go elsewhere.

For both IVF and ICSI, the cells are placed in an incubator to mimic the temperature of the human body and are observed closely. Some days later, the embryo will be transferred into the intended parent's uterus via a catheter. This procedure is carried out with the assistance of ultrasound while the recipient is fully conscious. The process takes only a few minutes. A pregnancy test is usually conducted a couple of weeks after the embryo transfer.

Any other embryos considered viable are frozen and stored for future attempts. In some instances, all of the embryos are frozen for potential future transfer. This is known as a 'freeze-all' cycle and might occur if the intended parent has vaginal bleeding or is unwell, or if the intended parent wants the embryos to be tested.

> ***Note:*** When donor sperm is used, most clinics will not allow you to 'bank' or freeze all of your embryos unless there is a medical reason for it, because it uses up a donor allocation. (For more information about Australian family limits see Chapter 9, 'Choosing Your Donor[s]'.) If it is your intention to bank embryos, check with your clinic whether it is a possibility before you start the process.

The IVF process is suited to people who have fertility problems (such as endometriosis or blocked fallopian tubes). It is also suited to people who wish to use frozen donor sperm.

Many clinics do not allow people who are forty years or older to undertake IUI, so IVF or ICSI may be the only options available for people over forty. Some clinics take this a step further and only allow people using donor sperm to undergo ICSI (see 'ART success rates' in Chapter 7).

Fresh versus frozen embryo transfer

What's the difference between a fresh embryo transfer and a frozen embryo transfer? The differences are discussed on the following pages.

Fresh embryo transfer

Prior to the development of egg-freezing technologies in 2004, fresh embryo transfers were the only option available for people undergoing ART treatment. As the name suggests, fertilisation is attempted immediately following egg retrieval—with fresh, rather than frozen, eggs.

How does it work?

The contraceptive pill is often used to synchronise the recipient's cycle with the donor's menstrual cycle. When the two cycles are 'in sync', the recipient commences a hormone regime to thicken the lining of their uterus and create the right environment for an embryo to implant. The egg donor commences medication to stimulate their ovaries and encourage more follicles to develop into mature eggs.

The donor then undergoes the process of egg collection (usually performed under light sedation or a general anaesthetic) while, at the same time, the intended parent's partner or sperm donor provides a semen sample in the collection room. Immediately afterwards, the donor eggs and sperm are prepared for standard IVF or ICSI. Upon fertilisation, the specialist assesses the quality and viability of the embryos created. A selected embryo is transferred into the recipient's uterus several days later while any additional viable embryos are frozen.

While the donor and the recipient are required to synchronise their cycles, they may never actually meet one another during the process because the embryo transfer takes place several days after the egg retrieval.

Undergoing a fresh embryo transfer with an egg donor can involve logistical hazards, such as: synchronising the availability of both the recipient and the donor; the donor passing the screening tests prior to each egg retrieval; and all of the complications (and expenses) that come with travel should the donor be located at a distance from the clinic.

Frozen embryo transfer (FET)

Once you have created one or more embryos, a FET cycle involves thawing one (or, in some cases, two) of the embryos for transference back into your uterus at the appropriate stage in your cycle. Frozen embryo transfers occur when gametes have been imported from other countries, when a person has excess frozen embryos following their ART treatment and when an intended parent is undergoing embryo donation.

Other instances where a FET cycle may be required include people who have polycystic ovarian syndrome in which the risk of ovarian hyperstimulation is high and it's difficult to align the cycles of the donor and recipient.

Frozen embryo cycles can be completed on your natural cycle without medication or using hormone preparations.

One benefit of using frozen embryos is that recipients don't need to undergo another full cycle of hormone stimulation to collect eggs (and, therefore, it doesn't cost as much). Recipients also don't need to be 'in sync' with their donor. Furthermore, donors are not required to be rescreened prior to each egg retrieval and the frozen embryos can be accessed at the convenience of the recipient.

What are the risks of IVF and ICSI?

Parents/Patients

The use of fertility drugs can, in some cases, result in ovarian hyperstimulation syndrome (OHSS), which is a risk for people undergoing IVF and ICSI (see Chapter 13, 'Being a Donor and How it Works'). Anaesthesia during the egg collection process can also cause issues such as nausea, vomiting and drowsiness, although the duration of the procedure is not lengthy compared to many other forms of surgery. There is the possibility of bruising around the ovaries from the needle puncture which can cause subsequent discomfort for several days.

In terms of ICSI specifically, there is a risk that an egg may be damaged during the process, rendering it unusable. Due to the process of natural selection between the egg and the sperm being taken away by the medical intervention, there is also a small risk that the sperm selected by the embryologist may have a chromosomal or genetic abnormality. This has the potential to impact fertilisation, embryo development, or lead to a child having genetic defects.[116]

With regard to the incidence of ovarian and breast cancer related to ART treatment, the jury is still out. While most studies have shown there is no increased risk, one Danish study looked at over 60,000 women and found that those who had undergone IVF showed a slightly higher rate of cancer diagnoses, although the study was unable to determine conclusively whether risk factors such as age also impacted the data.[117]

A 2021 study found that women who underwent ART treatment for extended periods (especially for more than a year) could be at greater risk, as well as those with a family history of breast cancer.[118]

Children

Research indicates that IVF and ICSI introduce a slightly increased risk of premature birth, still birth, low birth weight or multiple births.[119] A 2020 study concluded that the risk of pre-term birth (defined as below 37 weeks) in single pregnancies achieved following IVF or ICSI was more than double the risk for naturally conceived births, although it was acknowledged that the cause might be multi-factored and more research is needed.[120] Another potential risk of IVF is multiple births due to the transfer of more than one embryo. Due to this risk, Australian clinics are regularly audited to ensure the incidence of multiple pregnancies is minimised[121] and, as a result, the number of multiple births has declined over the last decade.[122] Transference of multiple embryos carries with it an increased risk of premature birth, gestational diabetes and high blood pressure.[123]

Perhaps of greater concern is a 2018 study which suggested that children born after ART treatment are at an increased risk of birth defects compared with those conceived naturally.[124] More research is needed but, if your clinic insists on ICSI and you don't wish to proceed, choose another clinic.

Embryo donation

If donor embryos are being used, the intended parent does not need to undergo egg retrieval. The procedure is relatively simple and involves cycle tracking to determine when ovulation occurs. Then the embryo is transferred at the appropriate time, in the same manner as it would be for a person undergoing a frozen embryo transfer (FET) cycle [see 'Frozen embryo transfer (FET)' earlier in this chapter]. If the intended parent does not have functioning ovaries, or the lining of the uterus requires further preparation to make it ready for pregnancy, hormone treatment may be used.

Partner or reciprocal IVF

Partner IVF or 'egg sharing' involves one partner providing the egg, a sperm donor fertilising the egg and the other partner being the gestational parent. This is an alternative chosen by some LGBTQIA+ couples and means that both partners can be physically involved in conception and potentially experience a greater emotional and spiritual connection with their donor-conceived child. If you are considering this option, check with your clinic to ensure it is permitted.

Partner IVF is almost identical to standard IVF using a fresh embryo transfer, but it can also be done with a FET cycle. Sometimes the egg donor and gestational parent roles are reversed when a second child is wanted and, in some cases, both partners might be pregnant at the same time. Embryos can also be frozen for future use and FET cycles can be undergone at a later date.

Some people have reported that their Australian clinic's paperwork for partner IVF has not been up to date. This means that the person supplying the egg may have to complete paperwork identifying them as a 'donor', even though the process involves transferring their fertilised egg into their partner's uterus—this represents signing away legal rights over their child. It is obviously better for all parties that such a signed document does not exist! Make sure you address this issue with the clinic and insist on completing up-to-date paperwork only.

Further issues to consider are the significant cost of partner IVF, particularly in situations when IUI may also have been a successful option (depending on the age and fertility health of the individuals). Partner IVF also increases medical risk because both partners become patients of the clinic and both may undergo hormone treatment.

Trans and gender diverse people

What are the options for trans and gender diverse people when making decisions about parenting? As a starting point (prior to undergoing gender affirming medical interventions, if that is a consideration), fertility preservation is an option which provides for the possibility of using thawed gametes later. If, on the other hand, you have commenced hormone replacement therapy, it may be possible to work with a specialist who can assist in regaining your reproductive capacity and using your own gametes.

Some trans individuals continue to produce gametes despite gender affirming hormone therapy. So gender affirming hormone therapy should never be considered a method of birth control.

Trans men and transmasculine people

During the medical gender-affirmation process for trans men and transmasculine people, increased levels of testosterone are highly likely to result in the discontinuation of egg production and, potentially, of the menstrual cycle. Consideration could be given to conceiving a child prior to undergoing medical intervention. You may also consider undergoing fertility treatment to freeze eggs, or take it a step further and undergo IVF treatment to create and preserve embryos. Embryos could be created using a sperm donor if you are single or you have an egg-producing partner.

Even if you have been taking testosterone for several years, it *could* still be possible to obtain healthy eggs from your ovaries and create embryos.

If you have already undergone gender-affirming surgery that resulted in your uterus and ovaries being removed and you have an egg-producing partner, your partner may wish to be the gestational parent using a sperm donor.

Alternatively, if you don't have a partner with healthy ovaries, or a sperm-producing partner, or you have no partner at all, a donor (or donors) and a surrogate may be required.

Trans women and transfeminine people

The use of hormones during the medical gender-affirmation process may cause sperm production to cease so, conceiving a child prior to undergoing treatment could be considered. Otherwise, sperm could be frozen for future use prior to undergoing hormone therapy.

If you have already undergone gender-affirming surgery and have a sperm-producing partner, you may need an egg donor and a surrogate. If partnered with a person who produces eggs, your partner could conceive using your frozen sperm or sperm from a donor.

In all cases, when considering donor conception for building your family, ensure you discuss your circumstances with the appropriate people (your treating doctor, a counsellor, a fertility specialist and your family) prior to undergoing any fertility treatment.[125]

Gamete quality and treatment type

If you are using a clinic-recruited or international sperm donor, you and your fertility specialist will determine the type of treatment you undergo. The decision you make can impact your choice of donor. This is because vials of sperm are sorted into treatment types based on criteria such as sperm count. For instance, if you wish to undergo IUI (a treatment that requires higher numbers of motile sperm) and your preferred donor only has vials available for ICSI you will need to choose a different donor.

If you are using a known sperm donor, a sperm analysis may determine your chances of conceiving using ICI at home, or IUI at a clinic, or whether it would be a better option to undergo IVF (or another ART treatment). Depending on the options, and should you wish to keep costs low, you might decide to find a different donor.

If you are undergoing egg donation, the type of donor you choose and their location will determine which of the options—fresh or frozen egg transfer— is most suitable.

Quality of gametes

It's important to understand that, while clinic-recruited and international sperm and egg donors are screened to ensure they meet the requisite criteria, this does not necessarily guarantee high-quality gametes each and every time. In the following pages, we will examine some of the issues regarding gamete quality that need to be considered.

Sperm quality

> *The previous clinic I was using kept suggesting IUI when I had cancelled IVF cycles. My donor's sperm sample was even labelled, 'ICSI quality only' and a count of four million. Money making scam if you ask me. It was about $1000 a go and there was no way in hell it would work, and they knew it. I changed clinics.*
>
> **Australian recipient parent**

A sperm concentration of twenty million to eighty million sperm per millilitre of semen (give or take a few million) is considered normal.[126] Some counts can be as high as 200 million or more, while anything less than fifteen million sperm per millilitre is considered low.[127] To meet the donor criteria, a large proportion of sperm also needs to demonstrate good motility (forward progressive movement) and morphology (size, shape and appearance). Each sample collected at a clinic or sperm bank is usually divided into multiple vials or straws for multiple use, so a person with poor-quality sperm is unlikely to be accepted—although it has been known to happen.

A donor's suitability and availability for the range of ART treatments is directly related to their sperm quality and whether their sperm thaw successfully—in other words, a high sperm count isn't the be-all and end-all. For instance, donors with high sperm counts might be available for all treatments including IUI, whereas donors with lower counts or poor motility may, for example, only be available for IVF or ICSI. The treatment options for which a donor is available will usually be made clear on their profile.

The following information regarding sperm suitability provides a general outline only. Standards vary between clinics.

Intrauterine insemination (IUI) and intracervical insemination (ICI)

Of all the treatments available, IUI requires the highest sperm count. This is because, despite being manually placed into the uterus, the sperm still need to work to swim toward the egg and penetrate its surface.

International sperm banks usually guarantee a sperm count of ten to fifteen million per insemination, although some will proceed with as few as six million—and some with even less. Australian clinics might advertise their sperm quality and, in some cases, the advertised sperm count *could* be significantly lower than that claimed by international sperm banks.

Sometimes, if you choose to do IUI in a foreign country, they might insist you undergo multiple attempts. This *may* increase your chances of conceiving and will definitely increase the costs for sperm.

If you are using a known donor and undergoing ICI at home, completing a semen analysis prior to conception attempts could save you a great deal of time and money in the long run if your donor's sperm is shown to only be viable for IVF or ICSI.

In vitro fertilisation (IVF)

Given IVF occurs in a dish rather than in a human body—and the donor sperm have been separated, washed and prepared for treatment—less sperm are required for IVF than for IUI. During the IVF process, approximately 100,000 motile sperm are released into a dish containing a solution of culture media through which they navigate their way to the egg.

Intra-cytoplasmic sperm injection (ICSI)

> *My clinic let slip that they actually divide samples (possibly not all), which is why they are listed as ICSI and not used for IVF or IUI. They also don't do a full sperm analysis. I wasn't impressed. I wasn't allowed to choose a donor designated as IUI—they were making me do ICSI because of my age and they didn't want to waste the few donors they had that had sperm counts good enough for IUI.*
>
> **Australian recipient parent**

Theoretically, only one sperm per viable egg is required for ICSI, but the embryologist will try to isolate as many healthy sperm as possible before carefully selecting one high-quality sperm for insertion into the egg. This means that sperm from a donor sample containing very low numbers per vial could be used and it's unlikely that sperm count or quality suitable for ICSI will even be discussed with you.

Increasing your prospects of receiving high quality sperm

> *My first IUI they had trouble with the sperm. They ended up defrosting two straws with the sperm count being one million. They told me this number as I was in the stirrups. One million seemed like a big enough number but, once I got home, I realised this was not a great number. I complained to the clinic and they reimbursed me for that cycle and gave me the next IUI cycle free.*
>
> **Australian recipient parent**

Many international sperm banks advertise their sperm guarantees on their websites; in Australia, where clinic-recruited donors are less abundant and family limits significantly lower, clinics tend to be more restrained. Some clinics may provide all of the information about your donor's sperm quality quite literally as you're about to undergo treatment—an irksome predicament, indeed. The clinic may also advise you after frozen sperm have been thawed that motility is below their acceptable standards.

These concerns do not include scenarios in which gametes have not actually *survived* the thawing process.

The following are options for potentially improving your prospects of receiving high-quality sperm.

- Are you being proactive about identifying your clinic's standards for each type of ART treatment? If the standards are less than what you (or the current research) consider to be acceptable, have you voiced your concerns?
- Have you asked your chosen clinic (and international sperm bank, if relevant) to explain their policy regarding sperm quality? For example, in many cases refunds are only available for IUI samples or in instances when the donor's low sperm count has resulted in your treatment being cancelled.

- If there is a suggestion to change to alternative, more expensive, treatments because the selected sperm sample does not meet the required standards, are you willing to take the risk and pay the extra money?
- When an IVF cycle is cancelled due to your donor's low sperm count and a suggestion is made for you to 'have a go' at the less expensive option of IUI, are you willing to take that risk?
- Are you willing to accept the sperm bank's claims that your clinic or specialist has handled the sample improperly or read the results incorrectly (unless they admit they have)?
- Have you asked for a refund or a replacement vial if, upon thawing, the sperm sample did not meet the clinic's standards (or those of the international sperm bank)? If the gametes have been imported from an international sperm bank, your clinic can write a letter to confirm that the sample sperm count was of significantly lower quality than guaranteed.
- Are you willing to find another donor, clinic or sperm bank, if necessary?

Egg quality

While some obvious degenerative issues—such as a thick zona pellucida (the membrane that surrounds the egg) —may stand out to an embryologist, there is no single way in which egg quality can be measured. Certain tests can provide an indication. These include:

- an Anti-Mullerian Hormone (AMH) blood test, also known as the 'egg-timer' test, which establishes a person's ovarian reserve (the quantity of eggs they have remaining)
- a blood test to measure the levels of follicle-stimulating hormone (FSH)
- a transvaginal ultrasound to check the number of antral or 'resting' follicles on the ovaries. These follicles are immature eggs which could mature and be released for the current cycle.

While an AMH test may provide an indication of how many eggs remain and can assist specialists with determining the best course of treatment, AMH tests are not an accurate prediction of a person's *fertility potential.*[128]

Ultimately, the only way to know whether an egg is chromosomally normal is to fertilise the egg, then genetically test the embryo.

Increasing your prospects of receiving high-quality eggs

The following are options to consider for potentially improving your prospects of receiving high-quality eggs.

- Have you read your chosen agency or egg bank's policy regarding egg quality and subsequent promises? For example, do they guarantee a certain number of embryos created per eggs provided and, if no embryos are created from the first quantity, will they supply you with additional eggs for free (often referred to as 'a replacement')? If you are undergoing a fresh embryo transfer, are there any guarantees when the outcome is a small number of embryos, or no embryos? Alternatively, does the agency/egg bank make no promises at all?
- Have you asked the egg bank or agency about the donor's previous results, including the number of blastocysts created, how many were successfully transferred, how many were thawed successfully, the cycle outcomes and how many live births there were? The donor may have previously produced a large number of eggs without the result being a successful pregnancy. These details will provide you with a clearer picture of your donor's fertility than a number displayed on the egg bank/agency's website.

  And just because you choose a younger person as your donor, this does not guarantee they will produce an abundant supply of high-quality eggs, or that the eggs will be suitable to freeze.
- Does the egg bank or agency outsource their egg donor processes to local fertility clinics? If so, this *could* mean standards are compromised in areas such as donor recruitment, staff training and experience, quality measures and protocol around egg retrieval and freezing. Furthermore, when egg banks outsource their processes, instead of one direct shipment to your clinic, there is the potential for donor eggs to be shipped multiple times increasing the risk of them thawing.

- Have you checked whether the international egg bank *imports* gametes from foreign countries? Importation *could* again increase the risks related to donor recruitment processes, screening, vitrification and unwanted thawing, as well as the absence or unreliability of success rate data.
- Have you checked the egg bank or agency's advertised success rate and identified whether their claims of 'guaranteed success', 'proven donor', or other similar terms equate to live births and not just to successfully completed IVF cycles or other interpretations?
- What is the egg bank's replacement rate (that is, the frequency with which purchased eggs are replaced when a guaranteed embryo was not created)? If the replacement rate is high, this means you also have a greater chance of needing to start again with a new donor, waiting longer *and* paying for an additional cycle.
- Does the egg bank offer a refund program? A refund will not usually include travel costs, treatment cycle costs, etc.—so the offer of refunds is not necessarily something to get excited about.
- Are you willing to find another egg bank or agency, if necessary?

The cost of ART treatment and factors to consider

Prices can vary from clinic to clinic in the range of thousands of dollars, so it is definitely worth making enquiries at multiple clinics. It is also important to note that, while treatments are often quoted as an all-inclusive package, additional costs invariably arise (such as travel, diagnostic testing, medication, theatre and anaesthetist fees).

Clinics are ethically bound to provide an explanation of all costs, although a 2019 inquiry into ART practices indicated that information about costs is often poorly communicated.[129] This lack of communication might include inadequate information regarding possible fees and associated out-of-pocket expenses.[130] To avoid shocks later, make sure that before commencing treatment you have an in-depth discussion with your clinic about all of the possible costs, including out-of-pocket expenses and hospital bed fees.

Medical Infertility

Australians need to be deemed 'medically infertile' to be eligible for the Medicare rebate associated with ART treatment. This makes it challenging for many singles and LGBTQIA+ individuals and families to undergo ART treatment when fertility is an unknown. People who don't meet this definition are sometimes referred to as 'socially infertile' (a somewhat unflattering and base descriptor).

So, what exactly is the definition of medical infertility and what criteria does Medicare use to determine whether or not a person qualifies for the rebate?

The answer to that enigmatic question is that *there is no precise definition.*

How does it work?

Medicare will only pay for 'clinically relevant' services when it has been determined by a fertility specialist that ART treatment is necessary to 'treat a patient's medical infertility'.[131] In other words, as long as your fertility specialist has ticked the box, you will receive the Medicare rebate.

So how does one move forward with fertility treatment and this particular obstacle without remortgaging the house? While some specialists might advise patients upfront that there is no Medicare rebate available and only offer a full-fee service, many will try hard to help you by assessing your fertility. Tests might include pelvic ultrasounds and checking your ovarian reserve (how many eggs you have remaining) and if, for example, you are very low on eggs, have irregular periods or have endometriosis, you may be eligible. This also means, perhaps ironically, that the likely treatment proposed to address your infertility will be IVF, a significantly more expensive option than IUI.

Another option presented by some clinics is for you to undergo IUI a couple of times and, if you don't conceive, this may tip you into the medically infertile category where, again, you will need to complete IVF. For heterosexual couples, trying to conceive for twelve months without success will get you over the line.

There are severe penalties for specialists who breach Medicare's guidelines.[132]

In all situations, ensure you discuss medical infertility with your specialist upfront (before you decide on a treatment option), so you do not receive a post-fertility-treatment letter from Medicare, indicating that no welcome credit will be landing in your bank account. If you believe you qualify as medically infertile and your specialist disagrees, you have every right to find a different specialist.

> ***Note:*** Eligibility to access ART treatment *may* be expanded in the future to include anyone who is unable to conceive without access to an ART procedure. Furthermore, if a person is not eligible for the Medicare rebate, that amount *may* also be covered by public egg and sperm banks.

Medicare

Who is 'the patient' for the purposes of the Medicare rebate?

Before proceeding with ART treatment, check your own eligibility for the Medicare rebate, then check the eligibility of your partner (if that applies) and, if you are using a known donor, ensure the donor has a valid Medicare card.

For the purposes of the Medicare rebate, 'the patient' is always the person undergoing ART treatment.

How does it work?

Clinic-recruited donors

In the cases of both sperm and egg clinic-recruited donation, the intended parent is responsible for paying for the costs of their own ART treatment and will duly receive any Medicare rebate for which they are eligible. The clinic will also charge a variety of fees to cover the cost of clinic processes and administration (such as recruitment, collection, screening and freezing of donor gametes).

Known donors

Likewise, when a person uses a known sperm or egg donor via a clinic, 'the patient' (for the purposes of Medicare) is the person undergoing ART treatment. If two people wish to undergo reciprocal IVF, both 'patients' will receive any Medicare rebate for which they are eligible.

In the case of egg donors, the egg donor is the patient, up to and including the egg retrieval process. The intended parent is responsible for payment of their donor's treatment and the donor signs paperwork to ensure the intended parent receives any relevant Medicare rebate. For the next step in the process—the embryo transfer—the intended parent becomes the patient and duly receives any Medicare rebate for which they are eligible.

If the donor experiences medical complications as a result of the cycle, depending on the nature of the treatment, certain costs might be covered by Medicare (for example, a public hospital emergency department), and by the donor's private health insurance (if they have it). If a pre-arranged agreement has been made, the intended parent would cover the remaining costs.

Some clinics may offer a reduced, flat fee for a treatment cycle—but this could mean the intended parent cannot claim the Medicare rebate. However, the end result and total cost may still be cheaper than a cycle at another, more expensive, clinic—even after the rebate has been paid. Make sure you check all of the costs thoroughly before making a decision.

International donors

When a person imports donated gametes from an international sperm or egg bank to an Australian clinic, the intended parent is considered to be the patient for the ART treatment and will receive any Medicare rebates for which they are eligible.

If a person travels to another country to use a donor, they are considered the patient and could receive the Medicare rebate for any ART treatment undertaken in Australia prior to departure. But all expenses in the foreign country related to the donor's ART treatment, the embryo transfer, or anything else, are paid for in full by the intended parent.

What is covered by Medicare and how does it work?

When undergoing fertility treatment, Medicare only covers certain aspects of the process, including (but not limited to) consultations, blood tests and ultrasounds. More complex procedures and add-ons are not usually covered.[133] If you ask your clinic to itemise all of the Medicare-eligible items involved in your treatment, you can calculate your out-of-pocket costs on the Medicare website.[134]

What is the Medicare Safety Net?

The Medicare Safety Net is an Australian Government initiative that means, once you reach a certain dollar amount for out-of-pocket expenses in a calendar year, Medicare will give you a higher amount back. Certain criteria must be met before you're eligible for the Medicare Safety Net benefit.[135] With regard to fertility treatment and the Medicare Safety Net, there is no limit to the number of cycles you can undergo.[136]

Concession cards

If you have a concession card—for example, Health Care or Pensioner Concession—in many cases, you will be eligible for significant discounts on medications. Ensure you mention your concession card to the pharmacist when collecting prescriptions.

Private health cover

If you have private health cover, check whether your policy and level of cover includes fertility treatment. You *could* be eligible for rebates when treated as an inpatient at a hospital—but note that having a procedure or consultation in a hospital doesn't necessarily mean you qualify as an inpatient.

Sometimes health insurers' policies have exclusions for some services and pharmaceutical products. Again, check whether the relevant item qualifies as an inpatient service or an outpatient service. It is a good idea to read the fine print on your health insurance policy or chat directly with a consultant. It's also useful to know that health providers do change minor inclusions from time to time, so check with them regularly once you know the names of the medications and other treatments you require. This could save you from receiving a nasty surprise in the form of a hefty bill at a later date.

If you don't have private health cover but wish to sign up for it, some private health funds consider infertility a pre-existing condition, meaning a waiting period will apply. So make sure you get onto this quickly.

And while giving birth may not be in the forefront of your mind at this point in time, it is also useful to consider how and where you would like to give birth and check whether this will be covered by your private health insurance.

Breakdown of costs

The cost of ART treatment can vary enormously between clinics and can usually be broken down into the categories listed under the following headings.

1 Cycle cost

This includes items such as scans and blood tests, as well as consultations with the donor team, nurses and fertility specialist.

2 Egg retrieval

Egg retrieval is normally completed under anaesthetic or light sedation, either in hospital or at a day surgery. This means there may also be anaesthetist's fees.

3 Gametes

The way in which you access and pay for your donor's gametes varies from clinic to clinic.

If you are using an egg donor, the only time you will be required to pay separately for gametes is if your clinic is importing frozen eggs for you from overseas. Otherwise, the eggs retrieved during the donor's cycle are included as part of the treatment.

If you undergo ART treatment at a clinic with a clinic-recruited or international sperm donor, you will pay a set price for gametes. Sperm from an international donor usually costs more. Depending on the clinic's policy and your success with becoming pregnant, you may have to purchase more than one vial of sperm (see Chapter 7, 'Choosing an Australian Fertility Clinic', and Chapter 8, 'Choosing an International Sperm/Egg Bank, or Egg Agency').

And, wait for it—not only could there be a cost to *join* the donor waiting list, you might also need to pay to *access* that list.

4 Specialist appointments

The cost of specialist appointments is also something that varies from clinic to clinic. In some cases, the first appointment might be free while, in others, ongoing appointments may be covered as part of your cycle cost. Or they may not.

5 Fertility medication

The cost of medication will be dictated by a number of variables including the recommended treatment plan, your current state of health, fertility issues you present with and, if conception is achieved, any ongoing requirements of your pregnancy. It is virtually impossible to predict how much of your hard-earned cash you may hand over to the pharmaceutical companies. Some of the medications may be included in the Pharmaceutical Benefits Scheme (PBS) and will be relatively inexpensive. If you have a concession card, they will be even cheaper, while others may be in a similar price bracket to 'cheap flights to Bali'.

6 Storage

Depending on your circumstances and the treatment being undergone, you will need to factor in storage fees for frozen eggs, sperm and/or embryos. Some clinics will provide one year of free storage, so make sure you ask about this upfront.

7 Travel

If you are undergoing part or all of your treatment interstate or overseas, you will need to factor in airfares, accommodation, airport transfers, travel to and from the clinic, meals and travel insurance. If your donor needs to travel to the clinic, you may also have to pay for their travel costs (see Chapter 7, 'Choosing an Australian Fertility Clinic', and Chapter 8, 'Choosing an International Sperm/Egg Bank, or Egg Agency').

The cost of intracervical insemination (ICI)

The basic elements for ICI include a needleless syringe, a semen collection kit, a sperm-friendly lubricant (lubricants can have unfavourable effects on sperm motility[137]), baby wipes and medical gloves. If your donor is travelling to your location to provide the donation, reimbursing the donor for *reasonable* out-of-pocket expenses is acceptable, although legal advice should be obtained to ensure no breach of the law occurs. Semen analysis and blood tests incur additional expenses.

The cost of intrauterine insemination (IUI)

If you undergo IUI at a clinic, costs will vary significantly depending on the clinic (different clinics could require you to undergo different procedures). Costs also depend on whether or not your procedure involves medication and how many vials of sperm the clinic insists you purchase. Some clinics allow purchase of one vial of sperm at a time, which could save you thousands of dollars.

Other costs might include a one-off registration fee, pre-treatment blood testing, ultrasounds and blood monitoring, counselling for yourself and your partner (if this applies), storage and the IUI procedure itself.

If you undergo IUI with your known donor at a clinic, despite not having to pay for sperm, the cost *may* end up being similar to what it would have been with a clinic-recruited donor, due to the need for procedures such as sperm collection and analysis, screening, storage and counselling sessions. Sometimes using a known donor could even cost more. On the upside, you might also end up with significantly more vials of sperm than you would have with a clinic-recruited donor and those vials are all yours to use.

The cost of IVF and ICSI

The most expensive of the ART options is IVF; and ICSI incurs an additional expense. Over and above the clinic's package quote, additional costs might include regular travel to the clinic for testing during a cycle, potential absenteeism from work, medications that are not covered by Medicare, and so on. If you are not eligible for the Medicare rebate, your costs per cycle will exceed five figures.

The cost of frozen embryo transfer (FET)

The comparative cost for FET cycles is less than for full IVF cycles and a cost is incurred for each cycle attempt. Storage of frozen embryos and sperm vials, if required, also incurs a cost.

Excess embryos

While the possibility of there being excess embryos should be discussed during counselling, conceptualising those surplus embryos (and what you might do with them) may not always align with reality—and the cogitation that follows . . . 'Oh, what to do with them!' . . . 'Should I save them in case I want another baby?' . . . 'Should I donate them to research?' . . . 'Should I donate them to another person or couple?'

More notable is the realisation that, should they be donated, the embryos will be full siblings to any existing children you might have, as well as half-siblings if donor gametes were used to create the embryos in the first place. This situation is often cause for significant disquietude.

Primary consideration when making a decision should be given to the donor-conceived children born from those donations and the potential impacts on their lives (see Chapter 9, 'Choosing Your Donor[s]').

Note: If an Australian clinic intends to collect your embryos, they must first discuss with you the options regarding the use, storage and discarding of the embryos (even if some options are not available at that clinic) and also allow you sufficient time to make an informed decision, including further counselling if required.[138]

Following is a list of some of the options for managing excess embryos.

- Store them at the clinic for the allowable period of time, at a cost. (Many people are forced into making a decision when the storage time lapses.)
- Apply to have the storage time extended until a decision is made (see Chapter 16, 'ART Regulations and Ethical Guidelines').
- Undergo a 'compassionate transfer', a procedure that involves placing the embryos back in your body at a time when you are unlikely to become pregnant.
- Donate the embryos for use in embryology training [for example, pre-implantation genetic diagnosis (PGD) biopsy training].
- Donate them to research.
- Instruct the clinic to dispose of them.
- Take the embryos home to bury or cremate—the ashes can also be made into keepsakes (such as jewellery).
- Donate your embryos to another family. When this option is selected, there may still be excess embryos after the recipients of your donation have completed their family or have given up trying—so you would, again, need to decide what to do with any remaining embryos.

Note: Not all options listed above may be possible if the donor does not agree, or the clinic does not allow it.

12

Conscious Conception: Preparing for conception and pregnancy with a donor

The 90–120 days before an egg is ovulated (or collected, if you're having fertility treatment) can significantly impact the genetic material you pass onto your baby, and their future long-term health.

Lucy Lines (Australian embryologist and contributing author to *Achieving parenthood*)

> ***Note:*** The information in this chapter is not intended to constitute health advice nor to act in any way as a substitute for consultation with a licensed health practitioner. Please consult with your own healthcare specialist before making important personal decisions.

When preparing for pregnancy, it's important to be aware that sperm takes about two months to reach maturity and that egg maturation, prior to ovulation, takes about three months. This means you might want to start thinking about matters a little earlier than first planned, to maximise the possible success rate of your conception attempts. It's also important to know that the *condition* of the egg and sperm at the time of both maturation and conception can have a lasting impact on how the genes express themselves and on the ongoing health of your child.[139]

But can we actually influence the quality of our gametes? A fair amount of research suggests that, yes, we can. While new sperm are constantly being created in the testes and can therefore be readily influenced during the maturation window of seventy days, the number of eggs a person has is determined at birth and only decreases throughout life; so eggs need to be considered on the basis of egg quality versus egg health. Egg quality refers to the DNA status of the egg and cannot be changed. Egg health, on the other hand, refers to the parts of an egg that can be influenced and changed—which can be achieved through diet and lifestyle.[140]

Conscious conception

Do you want to give your child the best possible start in life? All of us have within us an innate wisdom about the natural rhythms of life. Choosing a holistic approach to life (one involving mind and body), means you create a level of self-awareness that can profoundly impact your own life and that of your child. This involves preparing yourself before conception. Is your body in the best condition it can be? Are you eating a healthy diet and exercising? Do you meditate? Are you as stress-free as possible?

What of your donor? Do you know much about their lifestyle, or their health? Do you trust your clinic, your bank or agency, your donor?

Some people believe that conscious conception takes place at an even deeper level and involves an ancient wisdom integral to the wellbeing of our species. They believe that the egg and sperm must be allowed to make a conscious decision to choose each other in the natural environment of the body and that interfering with this process can impact the essence of any child born from the union.

Using a donor can make this approach somewhat challenging to achieve (unless you're undergoing artificial insemination). However, in all cases, if we prepare ourselves as best we can through education and healthy choices, we can bring a child into the world knowing we did the absolute best we could for our child in that moment.

Diet and lifestyle

When I'm getting ready to donate, I take it really seriously. Why wouldn't I? My diet consists of a banana smoothie for breakfast, a wholemeal sandwich loaded with spinach, carrot, avocado for lunch, then broccoli spinach, carrot and celery with two eggs for dinner. I'll eat one serve of red meat per week. I only drink water, and if I get hungry between meals I eat almonds. I take one supplement a day, and I avoid alcohol, sugar, fatty foods and caffeine.

Australian known sperm donor

Diet and dietary supplements

There are many fertility diets scurrying around cyberspace, each claiming to increase your chances of conceiving. Whether the information you read is accurate or not, the benefits of eating good quality food cannot be denied.

When considering your own or your donor's eggs, current research indicates that: vitamin D may be a factor in improving pregnancy rates;[141] green leafy vegetables are a good source of iron and folate; wholegrain cereals may contribute to endometrial thickness;[142] and, as everyone knows, fruit and vegetables (ideally organic or free of pesticides) are important for general health.

Folate is important for the prevention of neural tube defects, such as spina bifida. Folate supplements should be taken at least one month prior to planning a pregnancy.[143]

And what does your sperm donor or sperm-producing partner's diet look like? Are they committed to presenting you with the healthiest gametes they can muster? While more research is needed, there appear to be links between diet and sperm quality and, in some cases, positive changes can be seen in a matter of weeks. For instance, as well as consuming good quality food (such as vegetables, fruit, whole cereals, low-fat dairy and foods that are rich in fibre and antioxidants), improved sperm quality has also been linked to an increased intake of selenium, zinc and a handful of other elements. Furthermore, adherence to a healthy diet has also been linked to improved sperm concentration and motility.[144]

Consult with a health professional for advice on improving the quality or health of you and your donor's gametes.

Weight

Weight is a complex and sensitive issue and is not as cut and dried as eating less and exercising more. There are many factors that contribute to a person's weight including genetics, environment, hormonal changes, metabolism and socio-economic factors.

In the medical model, weight is seen as a major determinant of health, despite there being many factors that contribute to an individual's health. As a result, weight bias is a significant social issue which can also lead to weight stigma for larger bodied people. Moreover, an assumption is often made that a smaller bodied person is healthy, whereas a larger bodied person is not. When it comes to ART treatment, there are many reports of people being told to lose significant amounts of weight before they can undergo their next cycle, despite research indicating that dieting is not only associated with the development of eating disorders but is also linked to depression, anxiety and, ironically, weight gain.[145] Research indicates that disordered eating has been reported in up to 48% of women seeking fertility treatment.[146]

Furthermore, clinic-recruited and agency egg donors are generally required to have a 'healthy' body mass index (BMI)—however, it's important to be aware that BMI has repeatedly been called out as an inaccurate measure of health because it does not account for factors such as bone density, body fat, muscle mass, sex, race, ethnicity and, perhaps most importantly, a person's lifestyle.

Despite the existence of weight bias and inaccurate measures of health (such as BMI) studies have shown that the health of some larger bodied individuals can be at risk. Weight-related health issues might include interference with ovulation, a negative effect on egg quality,[147] the need for higher doses if stimulation drugs are required, and a subsequent increased risk of OHSS. Similarly, if your sperm donor or sperm-producing partner is a larger-bodied person, there *could* be issues with the quality of their sperm and reproductive hormones.[148]

People who are considered *underweight* may experience irregular menstrual cycles or can stop ovulating altogether, which then impacts their ability to conceive.[149] Some larger bodied individuals may also experience complications during pregnancy such as miscarriage, premature birth, gestational diabetes, and high blood pressure (pre-eclampsia). Babies of larger bodied parents are at greater risk of being stillborn or having a birth defect.[150] If you are smaller bodied, you may be at risk of giving birth prematurely.[151]

If your specialist is insisting you lose weight before commencing treatment, a question you might wish to consider asking is whether they can first assess other health markers before arriving at this decision. You might also wish to share any concerns you have about your body image, food and eating, as well as expressing to your fertility specialist that it is your right not to be weighed. Alternatively, you could seek out a specialist who is educated in eating disorder informed care to ensure you develop and maintain a healthy relationship with your body and avoid harm.[152]

Some people have reported being body-shamed by their health professional. If this happens to you, be sure to make a complaint (see Chapter 7, 'Choosing an Australian Fertility Clinic').

See 'Useful tools and resources' at the back of this book for links to online sources containing additional resources, blog articles and the latest updates, including a source for locating health practitioners at Size Inclusive Health Australia.

Exercise

How often do you exercise? Are you a couch potato or a fitness fanatic, or are you somewhere in between? Although everyone's body is different, evidence suggests that, when it comes to fertility, exercising at an 'in between' level is best.

Exercise has many benefits including improved metabolism and circulation— both of which contribute to better egg production and improved sperm quality. Exercise can also reduce stress levels, and evidence suggests that stress can negatively impact your reproductive system (see 'Mental health' later in this chapter).

On the other hand, some studies reveal that high-intensity exercise may actually reduce fertility so, if you are using a known donor, you might wish to consider checking in with them regarding their exercise regime.[153]

If you're not certain about how much exercise is right for you, speak to your health professional.

Alcohol

Research indicates that consumption of alcohol, even in very small quantities, has an effect on conception. For men and people who produce sperm, excessive alcohol can cause impotence and can impact sperm quality. Alcohol consumption during pregnancy (particularly binge drinking) can increase the risk of miscarriage, stillbirth, premature birth and Foetal Alcohol Spectrum Disorder.[154]

If your sperm donor is a clinic-recruited or international donor, the effects of significant alcohol consumption might become apparent during a semen analysis.[155] If you are using an egg donor, how many viable embryos have you managed to create? Could alcohol be a factor?

If you are using a known donor, do you know how much alcohol they are consuming? You might want to check how frequently your donor imbibes, just to make sure you're not wasting your time and money on poor-quality gametes that may negatively impact conception and your future child's health.

Smoking

The data related to smoking and fertility is fairly consistent: smoking can have a significant impact on conception and can damage the DNA of both the sperm and the eggs.

Is your egg or sperm donor a smoker? Smoking can cause damage to eggs and sperm and may impact the health of any children born.[156] Men who smoke heavily at the time of conception can increase their children's chance of developing childhood leukaemia.[157] If you are using a clinic, bank or agency donor, it is likely to be stated on their website that their donor selection criteria allows for non-smokers only, however this relies in part on honest self-reporting by the donors.

If you intend to be a gestational parent and you smoke, you have an increased risk of infertility and a poorer response to IVF; an increased chance of ectopic pregnancy and miscarriage; and, most importantly, a greater risk of harm to your unborn child if you do become pregnant.[158]

Are you a smoker? Did you know that the effects of smoking on gametes and fertility are reversible? If you're ready to quit, there are many different ways to achieve this.[159]

Caffeine

While, arguably, the most popular source of caffeine is coffee, it is also present in many other foods, drinks and consumables, including most teas, some soft drinks, energy drinks, chocolate and certain over-the-counter medications. There is some evidence suggesting that excessive caffeine consumption can increase the time taken to conceive and can also contribute to miscarriage.[160]

How much caffeine do you consume? Do you know whether your donor is a coffee drinker, or consumes energy drinks for breakfast? It's probably worth finding out.

Medication, including herbs and essential oils

Anti-depressant medication and other prescription drugs are fairly commonplace in today's fast-paced world. If you are taking *any* medication whatsoever, check with your fertility specialist to ensure your prescription is compatible with your fertility medication or your pregnancy.

Do you know whether your donor is taking any prescription medication long-term? If so, ask them to check with their health professional about the impact of the medication on their fertility and the health of your unborn child (or ask them for the name of the medication and check with your own doctors).

What about other forms of medication? Perhaps you ingest Chinese herbs for a chronic ailment, or you frequently indulge in a relaxing candlelit bath filled with essential oils. Herbs and oils may seem innocuous but they can be quite potent—especially when used undiluted. Some are considered unsafe during pregnancy. Make sure you consult your health practitioner if you are using any medications, herbs or essential oils.

Recreational drugs

Many recreational drugs can negatively impact an individual's reproductive system. Some can also increase the risk of miscarriage and stillbirth, as well as cause birth defects and intellectual disabilities in the children born. Depending on the drug, babies may also suffer drug withdrawal symptoms at birth.[161]

Do you know whether your donor is partaking in recreational drugs? If so, is it worth considering another donor?

Sexually transmitted infections (STIs)

Left untreated, sexually transmitted infections (STIs), including chlamydia, gonorrhoea, genital herpes, human immunodeficiency virus (HIV) and syphilis, can impact fertility. Some STIs can damage fallopian tubes, while others may increase the risk of miscarriage and stillbirth.[162]

If you have a history of STIs, speak to your health practitioner before trying to conceive. If you are using a known donor or a donor selected via a social media site, ensure you have a frank conversation about your donor's sexual health history. Ask them to provide you with a recent STI check (bearing in mind that it's only as useful as their last sexual encounter) or, even better, both of you undergo appropriate screening prior to your conception attempts.

Mental health

If you have been diagnosed with a mental illness (or believe you have mental health issues), it is important to consult your health professional prior to attempting to conceive. The process of conception, pregnancy and, most of all, parenting can be mentally, emotionally and physically challenging at the best of times. Your health professional can offer advice on how to manage these life changes, as well as advice regarding any medication you may be taking.

What about your donor? Are you aware of their mental health history and of their family's history? Can they, and will they, present you with a complete history for themselves and their family so that you can make an informed decision?

Stress

When it comes to fertility, research suggests that stress may be an issue for the health of both sperm[163] and eggs.[164] In some cases, stress can cause amenorrhea (the absence of menstrual periods) which is an obvious problem in itself but, primarily, stress upsets the balance of hormones in your body and can have a direct effect on your reproductive hormones.[165] To add insult to injury, if you are already stressed, the process of trying to conceive can increase your stress levels even further.

So, what can you do to manage your stress levels? Here are some suggestions:

- meditation and yoga
- moderate exercise
- ask for support from family and friends
- use the services of counsellors, healers and support groups
- practise asking for help (this will come in handy when you become a parent)
- practise saying 'No' to people who don't serve your higher purpose, or when you think you *should* do something (this will also come in handy when you become a parent)
- take a holiday or have a short break from work, if possible.

Environmental considerations

What about chemicals? How do they impact fertility and pregnancy?

Technically, *all* matter is made up of chemicals—the air we breathe, liquids, solids and, yes, our own remarkable bodies. So, what's the problem?

Rapid industrialisation has seen the introduction of thousands of new artificial chemicals, including a category of chemicals known as endocrine-disrupting chemicals (EDCs). Like other chemicals, EDCs do occur naturally in our environment but some of the artificial forms, such as Bisphenol A (BPA) and parabens, are present in pre-packaged food, on the lining of food cans, in food that's been sprayed with pesticides, on shiny sales dockets, in skincare and hair products, and in many, many other products.

Endocrine-disrupting chemicals are problematic for humans in many ways but, in terms of fertility, they can have negative impacts on sperm and egg health, resulting in pregnancy taking longer to achieve and increasing the risk of miscarriage. Furthermore, people who show high levels of certain EDCs often have less success achieving a pregnancy when undergoing ART treatments.[166]

What about your donor? What kind of cleaning products do they use? Are they inhaling toxic fumes on a daily basis? Is their work environment a safe place to inhabit for forty hours a week?

It's not possible to eliminate toxicity from our lives completely, nor is it necessarily possible to identify whether your donor is exposed to any of these potential risks—so what can you do? You can check your donor's career status and check their hobbies. Are they repeatedly exposed to spray paint, pesticides and herbicides? Do they drink from plastic bottles or eat a lot of pre-packaged processed foods and/or take-away foods? Do they regularly apply nail polish? If you are using a known donor, you can ask these questions directly, as well as more personal questions about their lifestyle.

Of course, you need to check your own level of exposure to EDCs. Is there anything you can do to make a difference to your fertility health?

Sleep

Did you know that your fertility is impacted by the quality, duration and timing of your sleep? Shift workers, in particular, can experience suppression of production of melatonin—a hormone that regulates your natural sleep–wake cycle and which is present in higher levels at night-time.[167] This reduction in melatonin can result in issues such as early miscarriage and failed embryo implantation.

Have you considered your sleep habits? Are you getting enough quality sleep? Is your donor? Is it time to consider all of the ways in which you can improve your sleep patterns? For instance, do you sleep with your phone next to your ear or stare at a screen right up until you go to bed? Do you eat dessert, or drink coffee or alcohol, late at night? Do you go to bed and wake up at significantly different times each day?

Contraception

If you are currently using contraception, check with your fertility specialist regarding when to cease taking any birth control medications or remove the contraceptive device—some contraceptive medication can take a considerable amount of time to cease being effective.

Dentist

How healthy are your teeth? While the old wives' tale of losing a tooth for every baby born is not so accurate these days (although still possible), some people do experience dental problems during pregnancy. The change in hormones can cause gum disease and tooth decay and, given severe gum disease is linked to premature births and low birth weight, it may be a good idea to see your dentist prior to attempting conception.[168]

Ovulation tracking

How familiar are you with the ins and outs of your menstrual cycle? Do you know when you are ovulating? Are you familiar with your fertile window? Ovulation predictor kits can help with this and involve a simple urine test.

Fertility specialists may recommend you keep a menstrual diary for several months prior to attempting conception with a donor. Smartphone apps are useful if that type of thing appeals to you. If you are unable to identify the signs of ovulation, seek advice from your health professional.

If you are undertaking insemination at home with a known donor, tracking your ovulation is vital to your chances of success. Is your donor available 'on call' to provide you with a sperm sample when your body is ready? Are you able to communicate freely with them and keep them informed of the probable timeframes? What if your timing interferes with your donor's social life and you are offered sperm that has recently been subjected to large quantities of alcohol? What if your donor has just spent a romantic weekend with their partner, or a new partner which may affect viable sperm levels?

Although you may be able to work out when you are ovulating, perhaps it is worthwhile outlining some criteria with your donor regarding what you consider to be acceptable and what you don't.

Where to go for help

> *I honestly don't know if it's harder to give up, or harder to keep going.*
>
> **Australian recipient parent**

When attempting to have a child, when is enough 'enough'? At what point does the cost factor—emotionally, mentally, physically and financially—simply become too much to bear? How do you make that decision?

If you are struggling to conceive or achieve a live birth, don't feel you need to suffer alone. There are many avenues of support available to you. If you are using a clinic-recruited or international donor, the clinic will have counsellors available to discuss your concerns. If you don't wish to talk to a counsellor (or you don't have the money to pay for one), there are online forums and support groups for people experiencing issues similar to yours. However, it's important to be aware that, while social media can be extremely helpful, sometimes these types of unregulated forums can result in further trauma by either dragging you down into other people's grief or ripping your heart into little pieces as a result of others' successes.

You might also have your own counsellor, healer, spiritual guide or support person that you can turn to if you need help. Perhaps you have an extremely supportive partner, or friends and family who can help you. Remember too that, if you have a partner, they may also need support.

In any event, there is no need to traverse the conception superhighway alone.

See 'Useful tools and resources' at the back of this book for links to online sources containing additional resources, blog articles and the latest updates about donor conception (including lists of organisations offering support, guidance; and the contact details of support groups for people experiencing infertility issues).

Part Five: All About Donors

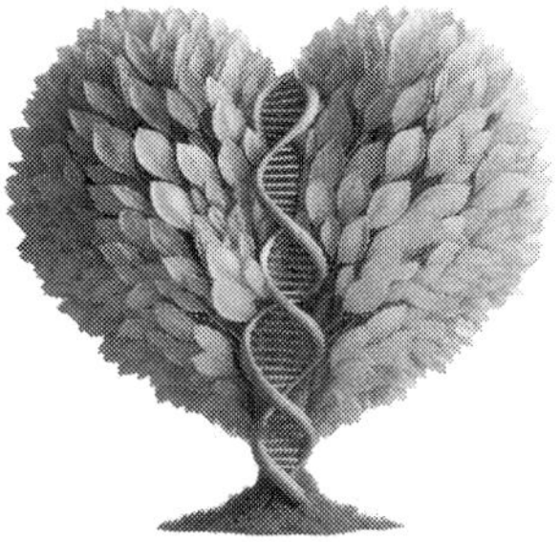

Being a donor has been such a rewarding experience. Being a part of a person's life story is a true privilege. I wanted to afford couples/singles the opportunity to have what I have with my beautiful children. I have donated to four couples, and have three donor children with more on the way. Each relationship looks different, but they all work, and I am truly blessed to be privy to their lives and watch them grow.

Australian egg donor

Depending on the type of donor selected, many recipient parents describe a kind of 'mental disconnect' between the *concept* of a donor and the reality that a donor too, is a human being with thoughts, feelings, hopes and dreams.

This chapter aims to provide you with an understanding of the range of feelings donors have about donating and what they might go through before, during and after the donation process. It also provides some suggestions for ways you might support—and in some cases, protect—your donor through your own choices, language and behaviour.

If you're not ready to read about donors and the donation process, skip this part and come back to it later.

13

Being a Donor and How It Works

In recruiting marketable donors, both egg agencies and sperm banks place advertisements listing biological requirements (e.g. age), but egg agencies emphasize the opportunity to help and sperm banks portray donation as a job, a distinction shaped by gendered stereotypes that appear in countless organizational processes.

Rene Almeling (American sociologist)[169]

While many, many donors are driven by altruistic intentions, the fact is that donor conception is a multi-billion-dollar industry. The marketing strategies rolled out by US sperm banks sometimes use blatant cash-driven phrases to attract donors, such as, 'Get paid for what you're already doing!' or 'Earn up to $1400 per month!' Sometimes phallic images are used, or references to masturbation with an assortment of euphemisms.

When it comes to international egg donors, the marketing pitches have also included statements such as, 'I just made $15,000 by donating my eggs!', or 'Donate your eggs and 'give up your day job'/'travel the world'/'take yourself on a shopping spree'! Then there's the approach that suggests your eggs aren't your own—instead, they're part of a larger gene pool spanning generations and geographic locations and you're just giving up another period.[170] Alternatively, a softer approach proposes that this 'wonderful gift' which requires 'a very caring person' will be 'life-enriching', and so on.

Some clinics (more so in countries like Australia where donors are reimbursed as opposed to being paid, and may already have a family) take a slightly more constrained approach to their marketing attempts, depicting sperm donors as heroes and tending to use images of brawny-looking men in speedos or firefighting uniforms. Advertisements for altruistic egg donation, again, share messages about generosity and the gift you'll be giving to families in need. Radio campaigns are also popular in Australia and there have even been accounts of people dressed as giant sperm handing out business cards in cafes. (Yes, that's right.)

Why do people become donors?

> *As a donor, it's difficult to conceptualise what it's going to be like for your donor-conceived child but, when I met my daughter, it was a primal feeling; the familiarity, the connection. You're passing on big parts of yourself to your child.*
>
> **Australian sperm donor**

Marketing pitches aside, what *does* actually motivate people to offer their gametes to others—strangers in most cases—for the purposes of creating children?

Again, the answers to this question vary significantly. At the altruistic end of the spectrum, some people are simply happy to help others create a family. They may have experienced infertility themselves and understand the heartache of multiple failed attempts, or they may wish to support those who are unable to conceive without the assistance of donated gametes. For some, being approached by a friend or family member to be a donor is the first time they have even considered the possibility.

From a practical perspective, many people find themselves in the position of having excess eggs and embryos after their ART treatment cycles and are then forced to make a decision regarding their use. One choice is to donate. At the other end of the donation spectrum, are the self-titled, 'super sperm donors' [serial donors] (see Chapter 6, 'Known

Donors'). Then there are those 'in-demand' egg donors with desirable traits, such as model-like features and an Ivy League education, who routinely earn five-digit compensation for their donations.[171] And then there's everything in between.

As well as helping others, some of the other reasons people donate their gametes include: the ability to have their own children where it is not otherwise possible (for example, in the cases of gay men); and the impulse to create a child for someone else and not 'let their gametes go to waste', while acknowledging a lack of desire to have a child of their own.

When it comes to known donors specifically, some of the reasons include: the ability to select their own recipients and get to know them before making a decision; the ability to connect with their children and influence their lives; to help recipients avoid the prohibitive costs of ART treatment at a clinic; fear of a clinic using their gametes for procedures without their consent; avoiding time-consuming recruitment, screening and counselling processes; not meeting the clinic's donor criteria.

Eligibility criteria

Australian clinic-recruited sperm and egg donors

Each clinic has its own set of criteria, and there is some regulation (see Chapter 16, 'ART Regulations and Ethical Guidelines') but, generally speaking, donors can be of any cultural, religious or ethnic background.

Health and lifestyle

Donors need to be in good health, with no evidence or history of illness or disease. Donors are also required to provide their family's medical history to check for the presence of genetic conditions that may be passed on to a child. Adoptees and donor-conceived people can only donate if they know their full genetic origins and history. This, of course, relies on the fact that an individual is aware of their conception story.

Donors (particularly egg donors) are *usually* required to be within a healthy weight range, according to the clinic's criteria.

Some of the reasons a person might be ineligible to donate include having previously been imprisoned, physical or mental illness, being a recipient of an organ transplant, and lifestyle choices such as smoking or drugtaking.

So, while all of this might sound terrific, it's important to know that many of these are self-reported and rely on the donor's honesty.

Previous donations

Clinics will not usually accept people who have previously been a known sperm donor. This is because there are no formal records of their existing donor-conceived children and the donor may have exceeded their family limit. The potential risk of this scenario is that an intended parent may create frozen embryos with the donor and then find themselves in the position of being unable to use them.[172]

Completion of family

Some Australian clinics have a requirement that egg donors have completed their own family prior to becoming a donor. This is because, unlike sperm donation, donating eggs is an invasive procedure involving drugs and surgery that may, in some circumstances, impact a person's health and in extreme circumstances render them infertile.

Most clinics also recommend that egg donors complete breastfeeding their existing children because the medications required during the donation process can reduce or stop milk supply. People who have had hysterectomies may still be eligible to donate, as long as they have functioning ovaries.

Donors may also be ineligible if they are in the process of undergoing ART treatment themselves; if their partner is currently pregnant; or if their youngest child is not yet twelve months of age.

Residency status

Donors are not required to be permanent Australian residents (see Chapter 9, 'Choosing Your Donor[s]').

Age

Sperm donors must be at least eighteen years of age (or up to twenty-three in some instances) and in *most* cases, no older than forty-five—although some clinics may set the upper age limit slightly lower or higher.

The limits for egg donors are generally capped at a younger age—usually around twenty-one (or twenty-three in some instances) to age thirty-five, due to the declining egg quality experienced by women in their mid-thirties. When a person is donating leftover frozen eggs, eligibility is usually determined by the date of egg collection.

The ages of eligible embryo donors vary between clinics and can also vary between the two people who created the embryo. For instance, some clinics may place the age of the egg donor between eighteen years and thirty-five years of age and the age of the sperm donor between eighteen years and forty-five, and, again, these age limits apply at the time the embryos were created.

When a person is using a known sperm or egg donor and undergoing ART treatment at a clinic, the age limit can be higher, as long as the recipient understands the possible implications (see Chapter 9, 'Choosing Your Donor[s]'). Check with your clinic regarding the rules which apply in that jurisdiction.

Partner consent

Clinics encourage donors to include spouses or de facto partners in discussions about donating, including topics such as the benefits of open disclosure and the potential impacts on the partner and on the couple's relationship.[173] Clinics rely on the donor's honesty as to whether they have a partner or not.

International sperm and egg donors

While most of the criteria for international donors will be similar to those for Australian clinic-recruited donors, each country (and each sperm/egg bank or agency) will have its own list of screening tests and rules, and these will usually be displayed on their website. As is true for Australian donors, much of the information is self-reported. Generally speaking, when donors are paid, more people tend to apply, the criteria are tougher to fulfil, and the percentage of donors accepted is considerably lower. Nevertheless, it's important to be aware that this does not automatically equate to high-quality gametes or honest self-reporting.

In countries where donors are paid, egg donors do not usually need to complete their own family prior to donating.

Known donors

When it comes to known sperm donors, the only criteria they are expected to meet are those stipulated by the intended parent. This applies to egg donors as well, but to a slightly lesser extent given that all egg donors are required to undergo ART treatment and will be subject to rules imposed by clinics. If you choose to take your known sperm donor to be screened at a clinic, they might also be assessed according to some of the clinic's eligibility criteria. If you are undergoing home insemination with your known sperm donor, the selection criteria are yours—and yours alone (see Chapter 9, 'Choosing Your Donor[s]').

What is the gamete donation process?

Australian clinic-recruited donors

If a person successfully meets all of the criteria at a clinic, they will become what is known as a clinic-recruited donor and be placed on the clinic's register to be matched with an intended parent.

So how does the process of donating at a clinic actually work?

At each stage of the process, the clinic will determine whether the donor meets the criteria and the donor will either be moved on to the next step or 'let go'.

> ***Note:*** The following steps provide a general overview only and may vary between clinics.

1 Expression of interest

The potential donor completes a lengthy and detailed questionnaire providing answers to a multitude of questions, including: their reproductive history; their lifestyle behaviours; medical history (*and* their family's medical history, along with an agreement to provide updates should new medical information become available), their ethnic background; whether they've had a tattoo or a blood transfusion; whether they smoke, drink or take drugs; and so on. When an embryo is being donated, the providers of both gametes need to complete the forms.

Depending on the clinic, donors may also be asked to answer questions that describe other aspects of their life, such as: personality traits; their favourite colour, favourite food and music; their skills and hobbies. They might also include a personal message addressed to the future child. This information is all passed on to the donor-conceived person at a predetermined age, along with the donor's identifying details.

Known egg donors who have connected with an intended parent via a matching site are also required to complete these forms, as are known sperm donors who undergo ART procedures through a clinic.

At this early stage, a discussion with a nurse coordinator/counsellor might also take place to ensure the potential donor is fully informed about the legal and psycho-social aspects of donating.

2 Donor screening

The donor then undergoes a series of tests including tests for: sexually transmitted diseases (such as HIV and chlamydia); blood type; and genetic screening for inherited conditions. The donor's partner is also required to undergo several screening tests.

If the donor is a carrier for a disease, this does not necessarily exclude them from donating and the risks would be assessed against the intended parent's status for the same condition. If a donor changes to another clinic, they may have to undergo the testing procedure again, because some clinics claim to have higher (or slightly different) testing standards than others.

> **Note:** It is possible for some people to have such low levels of the HIV virus that it cannot be transmitted through sex or childbirth, although people should always seek medical advice before proceeding with a known donor who has HIV. A sperm bank for HIV-positive donors is available in New Zealand.

Sperm donors

Sperm donors are required to provide a sperm sample to ensure their semen quality is of an acceptable standard for donation and to determine whether the sperm can survive the freezing and thawing process.

Egg donors

Egg donors are usually required to repeat the screening process prior to every egg retrieval. This might include blood tests to determine hormone levels and ovarian reserve, a urine test for drug screening and an intravaginal ultrasound to check the health of the ovaries.

Embryo donors

Embryo donors are required to provide data related to their genetic and medical health to assess whether there is a family history of inherited conditions. If either of the donors has an existing child with an inherited disease or disorder, the embryos will usually be considered unsuitable for donation.

3 Appointment with a medical specialist

A medical specialist will discuss all of the test results and family history with the potential donor to determine their suitability.

4 Appointment with the donor coordinator

The donor coordinator explains how the donation process works, as well as the legal aspects. The donor then signs a consent form which includes a declaration that they do not have an intention to claim parenting rights and that they agree to provide identifying information for any donor-conceived children once those children reach the required age.

5 Counselling

The donor (as well as their partner if they have one) must undergo counselling. If the donor is known to the intended parent, a group session may also be required which the donor's partner also attends.

Some donors have reported lying about not having a partner because they feel the screening process is time-consuming and would be invasive for their partner.

The counselling sessions might include discussion of topics such as: why the donor wishes to become a donor; the risks of donating; how being a donor might impact their relationships with friends and family; the importance of telling their own children and family; how the donor's partner feels about the donation; the long-term psycho-social implications for the donor, the recipient parents and any children born; and the rights and responsibilities of being a donor.

When an egg donor expresses a lack of intent to have their own children, particularly if they are very young, they may be subjected to multiple counselling sessions before the clinic is confident enough to allow them to donate. In some cases a final decision will be made by a board of directors or other executive body.

6 Collection process

Sperm donors

Donors attend the clinic on a regular basis for an agreed period of time (usually several months) and provide sperm samples for use by donor recipients. Unlike countries such as the USA, Australian clinics only collect a small number of samples before retiring the donor. This is due to the smaller family limits allowed in Australia.

The donor should abstain from drinking alcohol and avoid ejaculation for a few days before each donation, otherwise the sample may not meet the necessary criteria. Donors enter a small room, are provided with pornography and expected to masturbate into a sterile collection vessel. The donor hands the semen sample over to the designated person at the fertility clinic and provides confirmation in writing—every time—that the sperm sample belongs to them.[174]

Egg donors

Once an ID Release or known egg donor has been matched to a recipient, they undergo hormone therapy to stimulate the development of multiple eggs, followed by the egg collection procedure. In a manner similar to sperm donors, prior to donating, egg donors should abstain from sex (to avoid becoming pregnant) and from alcohol. But that is where the similarities end. Unlike sperm donors, egg donors must continue to attend appointments with the fertility specialist every one to three days to undergo ultrasounds and blood tests, as well as refrain from physical activities that might affect their swollen ovaries.

When an egg donor has been matched with an intended parent and is undergoing a fresh transfer, the eggs are fertilised and transferred to the intended parent several days later. The number of cycles an Australian egg donor may undergo varies between clinics and depends on the clinic's policies.

Embryo donors

A geneticist will assess whether the embryos are viable and suitable for donation.

7 Gamete screening process

Sperm donors

A semen analysis might be conducted every time a sperm donor provides a sample. A multitude of details are documented each time—including, but not limited to, sperm concentration (amount), morphology (size and shape), motility (the ability to move) and the number of straws created from the one semen sample (each sample is divided into multiple 'straws', usually for use with multiple recipients).

The quality of the sperm can vary for every sample provided and may be affected by factors such as smoking, drugs and anxiety.

Egg donors

There is no current method for testing egg quality and, other than obvious visible issues, the quality of an egg can only be determined once the egg has been fertilised. (For more information about gamete quality see Chapter 11, 'Assisted Reproductive Technology [ART], "At-home" Insemination, Success Rates and Costs'.)

Embryos

When embryos are created with donor gametes, pre-implantation genetic testing (PGT) is an option to consider but it does come with significant risks. The PGT process is used to test embryos and blastocysts for either a specific known single-gene condition or a chromosome variation.[175] This occurs prior to the embryo or blastocyst being transferred into the uterus and involves the removal of cells for biopsy. There is a small risk that embryos may be damaged during the process, so PGT may only be used in certain circumstances, including (but not limited to) selection against genetic conditions or to increase the prospects of a live birth. The ethics associated with PGT (such as differing perceptions and attitudes regarding conditions and abnormalities; and regarding the discarding of embryos) as well as the possibility of false positive and false negative results should be taken into consideration. Clinics must provide counselling for intended parents before they consent to this procedure.[176]

8 The freezing and thawing process

Depending on the type of donation, once retrieved, donor gametes can either be used immediately to create embryos (with any excess embryos being frozen), or the gametes can be frozen and thawed for fertilisation at a later date. The process of freezing gametes and embryos is known as vitrification and involves rapid cooling to prevent ice crystals from forming. This helps to preserve the genetic material and also improves the chances of the gametes thawing successfully. While a donor may present with high-quality gametes, the ability to survive the thawing process is also a critical factor for clinic-recruited donors.

Sperm donors

Once sperm has been collected and prepared for vitrification, it is transferred into vials or 'straws'. Usually, one sperm sample can fill multiple straws. The straws are then frozen, to be thawed at a later date. In some cases, a clinic might maximise the use of one vial by performing a process called scraping. This means that, rather than thaw the entire vial, a small amount of sperm is retrieved and thawed. This enables the process to be repeated later using the same vial.

Egg donors

In a similar manner to sperm, donated eggs can either be frozen following egg retrieval and thawed later to create embryos, or immediately fertilised with sperm to create embryos (which can also be frozen).

Embryos

Embryos created using donor gametes can also be frozen using the vitrification process and then thawed later for transfer.

9 Quarantine

Clinic-recruited gametes and embryos are usually quarantined for a period of up to six months. The reason for this is that some diseases are only detectable after several months. At the end of the quarantine period, the donor is retested for infectious diseases, such as HIV/AIDS and hepatitis, before the frozen gametes and embryos are released for use.

10 Matching process

Given the shortage of clinic-recruited sperm and egg donors, donors and intended parents are usually matched quite quickly.

International donors

The donor process for international donors is usually similar to the process used for Australian clinic-recruited donors (as discussed on the previous pages). However, depending on a variety of factors, the selection criteria and screening processes might be more, or less, stringent.

Known donors

When it comes to sperm donors, depending on the agreement made between them and the intended parent, donors can undergo AI at an agreed location (see Chapter 6, 'Known Donors'), or can attend a clinic to undergo ART treatment. In the latter case, the process will be similar to that experienced by a clinic-recruited donor (see Chapter 4, 'Clinic-recruited Donors'), although it *could* be possible for the clinic to release the donor's gametes without a period of quarantine if the intended parent is willing to sign a waiver stating that they accept the risks.

In all cases, egg donors are required to undergo ART treatment at a fertility clinic in a similar manner to clinic-recruited egg donors (see Chapter 4, 'Clinic-recruited Donors').

Known donors are able to make a very personal choice about who receives their gametes (see Chapter 6, 'Known Donors').

Risks of donating

> *There needs to be a reality check before donating and that means asking yourself: 'What's the likely outcome for the child?' And you may start off not caring about that, but I can almost guarantee you will later.*
>
> **Australian sperm donor**

Donors describe a range of feelings about donating their gametes.

Some people experience an incredible sense of fulfilment and gratification knowing they have helped another family; others express the sentiment that the world is a better place for having their donor-conceived children in it, or that it is an honour to be a part of their lives.

Some people don't think much about their donations for several years until they are triggered by an event such as having their own children. In this instance, they may wonder what has happened to the children conceived with their donation and whether they are being raised in a safe environment with parents who love and nurture them.

Those donors who have a relationship with their donor-conceived children often express happiness and delight at being able to share their lives with their children and, in many instances, with their own extended family as well. Upon meeting their children, many express fascination at shared genetic and behavioural traits. Some donors are happy to only see their children 'every now and then'. Then there are those donors who express indifference towards the process and disassociate themselves from the notion that the children are connected to them in any way, wanting nothing to do with them—ever. Conversely, some donors wish they had donated to more families.

In any case, it is not uncommon for donors to hand over their gametes without fully understanding both the short-term and long-term implications of their actions.

So, what are some of the risks involved in being a donor? These will be discussed on the following pages.

Physical health

> *I had mild forms of endometriosis, adenomyosis and PCOS* [polycystic ovary syndrome]. *After taking all the fertility drugs, they were very quickly debilitating and severely impacting my life for about 25–28 days a month, until I had no choice but to have a full hysterectomy.*
>
> **American egg donor**

While there are no physical risks associated with producing a sperm sample, egg donation is a different story altogether. Egg donation involves undergoing part of the IVF process, in a manner similar to what you would do if you were attempting to conceive your own child (see Chapter 11, 'Assisted Reproductive Technology [ART], "At-home" Insemination, Success Rates and Costs'). However, depending on the policies and ethics of the clinic, egg bank or agency, additional risk factors may be introduced.

In countries where people are paid, many gamete providers are lured by advertisements offering vast amounts of cash, without them fully understanding the potential ramifications of their donations. For instance, a study of 375 egg donors (86% of whom were paid) indicated that, while 65% of them felt informed about the short-term effects their donation could have on them, more than half of the donors did not feel adequately informed about the possible long-term risks.[177]

It is not uncommon for prospective egg donors to be advised that there is minimal risk involved in donating their eggs. And while studies on the long-term health effects of IVF patients do exist, there have been no equivalent studies regarding egg donation. One of the critical factors that has made research difficult is that clinics, egg banks and agencies don't make a habit of tracking the health of their donors in the years following their donations. The first longitudinal study comparing egg donation in the United States and Spain has been led by medical anthropologist Professor Diane Tober. This study is currently ongoing.

> *I was an egg donor in 1999 and I have had severe and disabling health problems ever since. I now run a support group for sick and former egg donors along with several other sick and former donors. Amongst the other donors I've met we've struggled with pain, neurological issues, endocrine issues, cancer, heart problems, diabetes, infertility, autoimmune disorders, and a number of other issues. The thing is, not everyone gets sick but, if it happens to you, there is no turning back and pressing the reset button. These issues appear to be permanent.*
>
> **American egg donor**

When it comes to donating eggs (and anyone undergoing standard IVF treatment), Tober divides the potential risks into three distinct categories as listed below.

1 Fertility drugs and their side effects

Possible side-effects to fertility medication include nausea and vomiting, diarrhoea, constipation, headache, shortness of breath, bloating, dizziness, mood changes, vaginal bleeding, pelvic pain, rupturing and swelling of the ovaries, and more.[178]

2 Surgical complications and reactions to anaesthesia

Some of the issues that can arise for egg donors after egg retrieval include reaction to the anaesthetic, heavy bleeding, pelvic infection, severe pain and dizziness.[179]

3 Post-retrieval complications

Ovarian torsion occurs when the ovary twists around its stalk, cutting off its blood supply. This constitutes a medical emergency. In severe cases, an egg donor may need to have her ovary removed. The risk of ovarian torsion increases with ovarian hyperstimulation syndrome (OHSS).[180]

Ovarian hyperstimulation syndrome, which occurs as a result of the body's exaggerated response to medication intended to stimulate the ovaries, represents a further risk to egg donors, and can result from a combination of excessive quantities of medication and poor cycle progress monitoring. Symptoms can range from mild/moderate to severe. On rare occasions, OHSS can be fatal. Complications include abdominal bloating due to excessive fluid retention, abdominal pain, shortness of breath, nausea, vomiting, blood clots and kidney failure. Egg donors who suffer from OHSS can be hospitalised for many days. Several different factors can increase a person's risk of OHSS; these include polycystic ovarian syndrome, being of young age, and having a low body mass index (BMI).[181]

Some countries, including the USA, are not required to report how many eggs are retrieved per cycle, or how many egg donors experience OHSS—this has the potential to leave egg donors vulnerable to not giving fully-informed consent due to the lack of accurate information. Eighteen eggs is considered high risk for OHSS but, in some cases, donors produce up to fifty eggs—some have reported producing as many as ninety. A scenario of this kind might occur when the clinic/agency is seeking a multiple-family, shared-cycle arrangement, as opposed to a single family receiving all of the eggs from one cycle of one donor. In some cases, the donor might not even be made aware of the shared cycle arrangement so will not have provided consent.

Shared cycles are less common in Australia and occur more frequently during a clinic-recruited egg donor cycle. Most egg donors in Australia are known to the intended parents and, given the intended parents are paying for the cycle, they also receive all of the donor's eggs.

> ***Note:*** Australian clinics and independent fertility specialists must provide donors and intended parents with accurate and timely information pertaining to risks. This should be in an easily understood format and should include information related to the risks of the drugs involved and their side effects.[182]

Clinics are also required to document serious adverse events in cases where harm, loss or damage has resulted in a person being hospitalised. These cases must then be investigated and corrective measures put in place for review at the next scheduled clinic inspection. Events which are even more serious, such as gamete mix-ups or a life-threatening incident, must be reported to the RTAC as soon after the event as possible.[183]

While this process seems comprehensive, the question remains as to whether all adverse incidents are actually reported in Australia and whether anything meaningful occurs as a result.

> *I've donated my eggs multiple times and once, when I was hyperstimulated and became unwell, they basically made out that I was just complaining. I'm pretty sure there was no report written about that.*
>
> **Australian egg donor**

While it is acknowledged that OHSS does occur in Australian clinics, a 2020 inquiry by the Health Complaints Commissioner into ART practices in Victoria indicated that adverse incidents, particularly OHSS, could be occurring more than the reports indicate and that there is a lack of transparency regarding those reports. There also existed a common theme in which people did not feel heard or believed regarding their adverse events.[184]

Refusal to hand over medical records

Australian clinics will provide donors with their medical records, but some clinics charge a fee.

However, there have been reports by international egg donors that an egg agency or bank refused to provide them with the medical records from their treatment cycle. This means they have not been provided with information regarding results of their genetic screening tests, dosages of medication administered to them, the number of eggs collected, and any other information about the treatment they underwent. The downstream effect of this is that a donor might not be able to supply their medical insurer with the information necessary to make a claim.

This, of course, begs the question *why* an egg bank or agency would refuse to pass medical information on to donors who were previously assured of a 'stress-free' and 'relatively safe' process. Furthermore, when an issue with the donor's well-being has arisen, such as the discovery that their own fertility has been impacted by their donations, some donors have reported being told that their records have been destroyed by 'flood or fire'.

Sexually transmitted infections (STIs)

For known sperm donors, in cases where conception attempts are conducted via natural insemination, there is a risk of the donor contracting a sexually transmitted disease from the intended parent.

Financial risks

Lack of accountability

In some countries around the world, where healthcare systems are limited or deficient, egg donors can risk the prospect of lifelong debt to cover medical expenses for debilitating side-effects resulting from their donation. In such countries, egg agencies appear to absolve themselves of all responsibility, refusing to respond to calls from the affected donor.

In Australia, a known donor may be covered by Medicare or private health insurance for some or all expenses (such as ambulance or hospital procedures) and might also make an agreement with the intended parent for them to share or cover these expenses.

Taxable income

> *The IRS taxed my compensation 45% and New York State taxed an additional 19% so, of the $5000 per cycle, $1800 of that went to me. Then factor in the expenses associated with three separate surgeries, all as a result of the fertility treatments. I won't get into the emotional impact of this, the irony of losing my fertility as a result of helping people with fertility issues, or the massive amount of time I lost with my kids because of the health issues of being an egg donor.*
>
> **American egg donor**

Depending on the country, payment for gametes is considered taxable income. For instance, in the USA, egg donors are usually classified as independent contractors and, in some cases, the taxable amount is as high as 50%. Sometimes agencies and egg banks forget to include this little detail in their sales pitch.

Child support payments

In Australia, known sperm donors who provide gametes to an intended parent who has no partner or spouse, depending on circumstances, could seek and be granted parenting rights, which might then result in the need for child support to be paid. In other words, a court will award rights and enforce responsibilities simultaneously. In such a case, a court would benefit greatly from viewing a preconception agreement. This is even more necessary where natural insemination occurred—although that's not the only factor and the court will consider what's in the best interests of the child.

One example of a donor paying child support when the child was conceived via natural insemination is the case of *ND & BM* [2003] FamCA 469.[185]

Note: All legal judgements are dependent upon a variety of factors and all cases are different. The judgment in the court case cited here will not necessarily apply to your situation.

Exploitation

Donor recruitment

> *I think the IVF industry would like us, as donors, to not think too much about the impact of what we are doing. If we did, we might walk away—and they would be left without the vital 'spare parts' that they need.*
>
> **Ian Smith (former sperm donor; 1980s [Vic.])**

In some countries, some clinics offer the option of a budget rate or a free IVF cycle if people agree to donate any eggs or embryos remaining upon completion of their ART treatment. In other words, a person who has never previously considered donating their gametes or embryos may find themselves tempted to become a donor for the sake of saving excessive amounts of money. This process may also have a devastating impact should the recipient parent conceive a child using the donor's egg or embryo, while the donor does not.

Marketing resulting in the recruitment and subsequent payment of young college students as donors is considered exploitative by many—especially when large numbers of donor-conceived children are produced. Tantalising monetary rewards, accompanied by little or no counselling, have been seen to result in significant problems for donors later in life when they develop some awareness of the long-term consequences of their actions.

Feelings of being used

> *As an egg donor I felt chewed up and spat out. With the exception of the nurse who called me twenty-four hours after egg collection, absolutely no one checked up on me. During*

> *one failed cycle, I was completely devastated and I felt like I'd failed everyone: the intended parents, my husband, my parents who'd been babysitting my kids. Absolutely no one checked up on my mental health—the doctor actually left me a message saying how disappointed he was. There is literally no follow through. All the counselling takes place at the beginning which is great, but where is the counselling afterwards? They care enough until they've got your eggs, and then that's the end of it.*
>
> **Australian known egg donor**

Some donors describe feeling thoroughly used by either the clinic, the intended parent or, in some cases, both. Others describe feeling like a machine that's just provided spare parts, a human cash cow, and various other expressions that align with being used and discarded.

Withdrawal of consent

Sometimes egg banks or agencies do not inform international donors about the health risks of egg donation until late in the donation process. Despite this, the donors feel pressure to continue because a match has already been created for them and withdrawal would mean letting the intended parent down. Other donors discover that their contract prohibits access to their medical records post-treatment and, upon seeking to withdraw, the sperm/egg bank or agency has revealed that they would be required to pay thousands of dollars for the cancelled cycle costs.

Withholding of information

International egg donors are not always told how many follicles are maturing and how many eggs have been collected. One cycle (particularly if hyperstimulation is involved) may produce high numbers of eggs which are then divided into multiple batches to be sold for thousands of dollars each. In some cases, particularly where donors are required to be anonymous, they are never even told how many children have been created.

Australian egg donors are entitled to know the number of eggs collected but, once the eggs have been fertilised, may only be advised about the number of embryos created if the intended parent agrees to share that information. All Australian donors are able to access information about the number and sex of children they have contributed to creating.

Psycho-social risks

> *I am a former anonymous sperm donor. There are conflicting emotions. The pain of having no clue where or how many biological children I even have is unexplainable. There is a feeling of loss. Do they even know they are donor conceived and if they do, do they give a shit about me? Do they hate me, do they love me? I would like them to find me while I am still alive and while my parents are still living. I am on every DNA website, on every Facebook page and the Donor Sibling Registry. I have no children of my own. There are days when I feel pride in that I did an honorable thing by fulfilling some couples hopes and dreams. There are other days when I feel I was being totally greedy and selfish for doing it.*
>
> **American sperm donor**

Fertility pressure

> *I was so invested in helping her* [the donor's friend] *get pregnant and felt so much pressure that I ended up seeing a psychologist.*
>
> **Australian known sperm donor**

Some donors describe feelings of immense pressure when donating their gametes, as well as a huge sense of letting people down when a pregnancy does not occur or egg retrieval is unsuccessful. Some egg donors describe a sense of shame and embarrassment when intended parents present images on egg donor matching sites of their hands (customarily scribbled on by the specialist) displaying the number of eggs retrieved, and describe the scenario as a competition—some describe having been hyperstimulated as 'almost like a badge of honour'.

> *Once an intended parent told me she was disappointed because she got sixteen eggs and only three fertilised. I had that sick, deep down feeling of letting people down. There's a lot of pressure and really high expectations on egg donors.*
>
> **Australian egg donor**

The donor's family

> *My donor-conceived children tracked me down via a DNA test and I hadn't told my own children that I'd donated. One of them disapproves of donor conception and was quite upset when she found out—the other doesn't disapprove, but neither of them want to connect with their donor-conceived siblings.*
>
> **Australian sperm donor**

Some donors report that being a donor has negatively impacted their own family later. This is particularly true in cases when donation occurred at an early age and no counselling took place. Donors, and their partners, who were unconcerned about consequences initially can change their minds when they realise that donating gametes has a much greater long-term impact than they first understood (or were led to believe). Sometimes partners exert pressure on donors to reject attempts at connection from their donor-conceived children, forcing them to choose between their relationship and the children. In some cases, the donor's own children might express disapproval of their parent's actions and refuse to have a connection or even acknowledge their donor-conceived siblings.

Furthermore, when donors keep their actions secret from family members, they risk being on the receiving end of surprised, angry, joyful (or other) responses from their own children and family members. This may happen at any time (in some cases, decades later) when family members are contacted directly by the donor-conceived children themselves or they find strange anomalies on their Christmas gift DNA test result.

Anonymity

In some countries anonymity is the only option offered to donors and all parties are advised at the time of donation that anonymity is 'best for everyone', and 'don't be selfish by attempting to make contact', 'you'll break families', and so on. Many donors discover later that this advice is erroneous and recognise they have unwittingly played a part in an industry narrative that does harm to donor-conceived people. Sometimes donors grieve the loss of the children they feel they have literally given away, with no way of finding them unless they undergo direct-to-consumer DNA testing.

Misrepresentation and broken promises

By recipient parents

> *Once I donated to a lesbian couple. After I'd handed over my sample, one of them shoved a twenty dollar bill in my pocket and said, 'That's for petrol'. Then they drove off and I never heard from them again. Maybe they didn't like me, or maybe they got a positive result? I suspect they were pregnant, because most people get in touch a few weeks later and ask for another attempt. I like to respect people's privacy, so I guess I'll never know.*
>
> **Australian known sperm donor**

A relatively common risk for known donors is for terms to be agreed upon but things changing when the child is born. A recipient parent, for example, might unilaterally decide to change the level of contact time that was agreed upon. A donor is then likely to feel disappointment that they are not invited to significant events such as birthdays or other celebrations if this was the initial expectation. This is obviously likely to have a devastating effect on the relationship between the parties. The donor might be left treading on eggshells in case they upset the recipient parents or, worse, might be blocked from all further contact. The recipient parent may inadvertently become avoidant toward the donor and the child misses out. Donors have described experiencing feelings of guilt and sorrow when they realised the recipient parents have no intention of telling their children they are donor-conceived.

By banks and agencies

Similarly, donors may experience regret when they have expressed a willingness to be known, but the clinic, bank or agency does not facilitate this request.

Rejection

> *One of my donor-conceived children made contact some years ago, at which time she was seventeen. She asked for family history and medical information. I shared that willingly—and too told her that I was open to whatever contact she may wish to have. I've heard nothing more from her. I find that sad—but that is her choice to make.*
>
> **Ian Smith (former sperm donor; 1980s, [Vic.])**

While many donor-conceived people experience fear about being rejected by their biological parent when they reach out for contact, the same fear is experienced by donors regarding their donor-conceived children. Will I get to meet my donor-conceived children? Should I make contact with my adult donor-conceived children? If I do, will I be invading their privacy and causing harm? What if they don't even know they're donor-conceived? How many children exist? Why don't they contact me? Will they reject me if I reach out?

Some donors describe the initial joy of connecting with one of their children, only to be told that the contact is a one-off and an ongoing relationship is not wanted. Others are contacted by their children with a request for updated family medical information only, receiving no information in return.

Being criticised

> *I once told a friend that I really wanted to get to know my donor-conceived children and he said, 'You remind me*

> *of someone who donated two dollars and wants twenty cents back.'*
>
> **Australian sperm donor**

Some donors who express their desire to know more about the donor-conceived children they've helped to create receive criticism from others: 'It's not your business' . . . 'You're just a donor—leave them alone' . . . 'You're invading their privacy.' These are just some of the responses donors can receive when they express an interest in their donor-conceived children.

Managing relatives

> *A parent of one of my donor-conceived children said, 'What is this bastard doing ruining our lives? He was supposed to stay anonymous.'*
>
> **Australian sperm donor**

Sometimes donors are required to navigate their way around awkward family situations. For instance, where multiple donor-conceived children exist in a family, one child may wish to connect with the donor while the others do not. This can create anxiety and can cause the need to tiptoe around conversations and meet surreptitiously.

In the case of known donations when the donor has a poor relationship with one or both of the raising parents, the child may pick up on the negativity and transfer this hostility onto the donor.

Sometimes donors who attempt to connect with their children are berated by a parent or other relative who had assumed the child's conception was going to remain anonymous.

Guilt

Some donors express sadness at not being able to play a part in their children's lives, understanding too late that their donation affected them much more than they had anticipated. Sometimes a donor might wonder if the person they have helped to create is safe or, in the case of known donation, may witness first-hand that the child is not living in a healthy and nurturing environment. Donor guilt can also be manifested from not being around for their children when they needed them, understanding that the role of donor as expressed by the fertility industry does not necessarily reconcile with the needs of the children created.

These are just some of the many experiences and feelings donors describe.

Donor rights and responsibilities

> *If a donor isn't prepared to accommodate the future needs of their donor-conceived children, they shouldn't donate.*
>
> **New Zealand sperm donor**

So, what rights and responsibilities do donors have?

The answer to this question depends on whether the issue is defined by legislation or policy, as well as one's personal perspective and opinion of 'rights and responsibilities'. For instance, something that one person might consider unethical may be considered entirely principled to another.

Legal parentage

For more information about legal parentage see Chapter 16, 'ART Regulations and Ethical Guidelines'.

The use and discarding of gametes and embryos

For more information on the use and discarding of gametes and embryos see Chapter 16, 'ART Regulations and Ethical Guidelines'.

Donor payment and expenses

In Australia it is illegal for a donor to accept payment for gametes or embryos (see Chapter 16, 'ART Regulations and Ethical Guidelines').

Australian clinic-recruited donors

Clinic-recruited donors are not required to pay for any part of the recruitment, screening or ART treatment process—all costs are covered by the clinic. Donors may, however, be reimbursed for reasonable expenses. A formal definition of 'reasonable expenses' has not been established so payments tend to vary significantly between clinics. Some egg donors have described their reimbursement as barely covering the parking fees when, for instance, the clinic is situated in the Sydney CBD. Sometimes the payments are made as separate reimbursement amounts and the donor needs to keep and submit receipts of all expenditure. In other cases, part payment is provided at the time of donation and the remainder is paid several months later when the gametes are released from quarantine. Sometimes a lump sum is paid at the end of the donation process.

Known donors

The expenses for known donors who undergo ART treatment at an Australian clinic are generally paid by the intended parents. Likewise, when known sperm donation takes place 'at home', any expenses such as insemination equipment or motel rooms would be paid by the intended parents. If your donor contributes financially to your ART treatment or in any other capacity throughout your child's life, this fact may be considered by the Family Court should a parenting conflict arise (see Chapter 9, 'Choosing Your Donor[s]').

International donors

In cases involving international donors, payment is defined by the relevant country and the bank/agency's policies. For instance, if a bank specialises in providing gamete providers who have academic degrees, the more advanced the degree, the more the donor is paid—especially if the college is Ivy League. Alternatively, when a particular demand has been specified by intended parents, such as a request for a specific ethnicity or very attractive features, donors may be offered (or may request) more money.

For sperm donors, payment might be provided for each sample that meets requirements. Some sperm banks pay donors an additional 'bonus' when a recipient conceives with their sperm. Other sperm banks pay what might be described as a salary if a person signs a non-compete agreement. This involves committing to a certain number of samples per week for a given period of time and only at that bank. Other banks might pay their donors monthly.

Some sperm banks offer donors periodic incentives such as gift vouchers and movie tickets for 'extra time and effort' (and, no, I'm not exactly sure how 'effort' is defined).

Payments for egg donors can vary enormously and, at the extreme high end, have been known to be in the six-figure range. In the case of multiple-family, shared-cycle arrangements, donors might be paid an amount for each recipient. In some cases, payments may increase for each donation cycle as a kind of 'past-performance-bonus' arrangement.

Donor IDs

Prior to the introduction of cryobanks, there was no such thing as Donor IDs or, in many cases, any data kept about donors *at all.* In today's world of donor conception, the donor is allocated a Donor ID and each clinic, bank or agency has its own unique identifying system. Donor IDs might be comprised of a few numbers or letters only, or a combination of both. Some banks also give donors an alias or a fictional name.

Sometimes donors are informed of their Donor ID; sometimes they are not. In many cases, a bank or agency will only provide a person with their Donor ID if they are still an active donor or, alternatively, the donor can view their own profile on the bank's website. Australian donors are usually able to access their Donor ID, but they might need to request it from the clinic. When company takeovers occur at international banks and agencies, records are sometimes destroyed. In other cases, the company taking over a bank might allocate new Donor IDs to the existing donors so that they align with that new company's operating system. Australian clinics are required to store all donor conception-related data in perpetuity (which relies on accurate data collection).

What does all this mean for donors?

In some countries, banks and agencies refuse to provide donors with their Donor ID or any details about the children born from their gametes. In other words, banks keep the donors anonymous, even to the donors themselves. In other cases, donors are provided with their donor-conceived children's data, but no Donor ID. For donors who wish to know their children's details or make a connection with them later, the lack of a Donor ID and/or any data makes it very difficult to investigate and locate the donor-conceived children on public forums and social media platforms.

Where Donor IDs are reallocated (in the case of company takeovers), donor-related data can be skewed because the donor has been assigned multiple Donor IDs. Existing data also has the potential to disappear. In some countries, people have been forced to take legal action to obtain their Donor ID when it has become 'lost'—again, 'flood and fire' disasters are not uncommon.

Sometimes donors and donor-conceived people wash their hands of inaccurate or unattainable Donor IDs and opt for direct-to-consumer DNA testing to find genetic relatives.

And perhaps, one day, donors might just have their real names displayed.

Telling other people

To avoid surprises, it is important that donors inform people close to them about the act of donating—especially their partner, children, parents and siblings. In this way, donors can address any concerns expressed by their family members. It also means there can be no shocks further down the track when donor-conceived people (or their children's children) attempt to make contact or, alternatively, the donor's adult children complete a direct-to-consumer DNA test and discover they have multiple siblings around the country or the globe.

In particular, telling a partner about previous (or ongoing) donations is extremely important. Partners can often feel uncomfortable about their role in the relationship, or the possibility of sharing their lives with donor-conceived people who are not genetically related to them. It can also trigger painful emotions if a person has not been able to conceive their own children but their partner is creating multiple children as a donor for other families. Any of these scenarios may result in the donor's partner vetoing contact with the donor-conceived children. In a 2012 online questionnaire involving 164 sperm donors, the responses from the donors who were partnered showed that around one-third of those partners expressed reservations about or opposed contact with the donor-conceived children/adults.[186]

Furthermore, many people do not factor in the *parents* of their donor at the time of selection, but many donors' parents express extreme sadness at discovering their child has conceived multiple children whom they cannot access. Contrastingly, there is also great joy expressed by those who do connect with their biological donor-conceived grandchildren.

Supporting your donor and preventing harm

> *Sometimes I feel like I was just a source of spare parts.*
>
> **Ian Smith (former sperm donor; 1980s, [Vic.])**

While the industry narrative might, in some instances, portray the person providing gametes as 'just a donor', many donors (and donor-conceived people) find this insulting—particularly when the donation was altruistic. Alternatively, in countries where donors are paid, some donors have suggested they felt like a 'breeding cash cow'.

It's important to acknowledge that donors are human beings with real opinions and feelings, many of whom experience harm (physical, mental, emotional and financial) as a result of donating their gametes. More importantly, research indicates that your donor-conceived child is likely to view the donor as a real person and not just someone who supplied some genetic material.[187]

So, what can you do to support your donor and, in some cases, protect them from harm? Following are some suggestions you might like to consider.

Language, promises and compassion

- ✓ Avoid using diminishing language such as 'just a donor', or 'they just supplied the egg/sperm'.
- ✓ Treat your donor with respect when discussing their role in the creation of your child's life.
- ✓ Consider your egg donor's feelings when announcing on public forums the number of eggs collected in a cycle.

- ✓ Do not provide a false identity to your known donor because you are planning to hide from them once your child is born.
- ✓ Avoid making false claims to your donor about allowing them to connect with your child once they are born.
- ✓ Check in with your egg donor after egg retrieval to ensure they are feeling okay—both physically and mentally.
- ✓ Demonstrate empathy and compassion if, for instance, your egg donor has become unwell as a result of their ART treatment.

While the following relate primarily to international donors, it's important to note that there are Australian clinics who have service agreements with sperm/egg banks and egg agencies that engage in some of the practices listed below. So you might consider this information when deciding whether to proceed with an international donor via your Australian clinic (see Chapter 7, 'Choosing an Australian Fertility Clinic').

General

Does the clinic, international egg bank/agency or sperm bank:

- ✓ counsel donors?
- ✓ treat your donor with respect and consideration?
- ✓ provide upfront honest and detailed information to people about the risks of donating, without downplaying the lack of research related to long-term health risks?[188]
- ✓ advertise and enforce reasonable family limits, so donors are not able to produce vast numbers of children?
- ✓ provide donors with data related to the donor-conceived children born from their donations?

Egg donors

Does the international egg bank/agency:

- ✓ provide donors' medical records following treatment cycles?[189]
- ✓ allow donors the option of signing up for only one cycle at a time?

- ✓ provide donors with the ability to withdraw consent without being required to pay for the cost of the cancelled cycle?
- ✓ ensure donors have full visibility of the number of follicles maturing during stimulation cycles, as well as the power to subsequently request medications be reduced?
- ✓ provide donors with the option of freezing their own eggs for free?[190]
- ✓ provide donors the option of being known, rather than persuading them to be anonymous?
- ✓ demonstrate a low incidence of hyperstimulation and reasonable quantities of eggs?

Known sperm donors

When undergoing at-home insemination with a known sperm donor, can you:

- ✓ communicate openly and honestly about your requirements for ongoing connection, if that is your intention?
- ✓ thank them for providing their gametes and keep them informed about whether you conceive and give birth to a child?
- ✓ maintain agreements about ongoing contact?

Donor support groups

Support groups (usually started by donors themselves) are available for donors—especially on social media although, predictably, many more egg donor support groups exist than sperm donor groups. Some support groups have regular face-to-face meetings and may even include recipient parents and their families.

Group purpose

Groups can vary significantly in their purpose and, while there is often crossover in discussions, some groups are quite specific about the types of donors that are permitted to join and the subsequent topics for conversation. For instance, some groups are set up for former donors who wish to discuss relationships with their donor-conceived children or ways of finding them. Some groups are for people who have had a negative experience (such as ongoing health issues) and require moral support. Other groups are established to discuss and advocate for change in the industry, while others may be set up with the express purpose of discussing ways in which to make more money or to find ways of getting around the screening process for issues such as mental illness.

Discussion topics

Like any group of people who come together to discuss a topic, the groups can run the whole gamut of opinions and emotions: people who are satisfied with the bank or agency they used; people who, conversely, want to 'burn the building down'; people who are happy about providing gametes; people who wish to make provisions in their will for their donor-conceived children; people who regret donating and want to warn others about their experience or about a particular clinic or specialist; people who share uplifting experiences about connecting with their donor-conceived children and families; people who wish to remain anonymous; and so on.

Oftentimes people discover that the 'low risk' involved in donating gametes, as described by their specialist, cannot be reconciled with the number of people in donor support groups who experienced harm. Some of the group discussions involve post-donation illness and how to recover.

See 'Useful tools and resources' at the back of this book for links to online sources containing additional resources, blog articles and the latest updates, including information about donor support groups.

Part Six: Talking and Linking

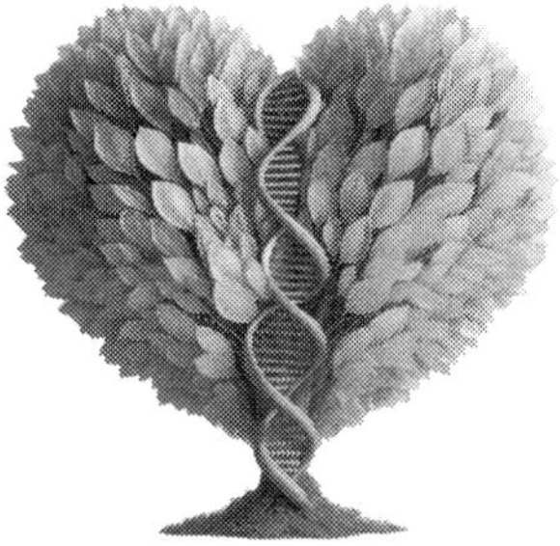

Recipient parents should be required to spend a few hours scrolling through pages like DNA Detectives.[191] *It's full of people looking for biological families. The need to know where you came from isn't unique to any group. Why would our donor-conceived children be any different?*

American recipient parent

The next two chapters describe ways in which you might talk to your child about their conception story, as well as the ways in which you can connect or 'link' with your child's siblings and the donor. Even if you don't have a child yet, these chapters can be helpful in preparing you for addressing the unique needs of your future donor-conceived child. The information may also help to influence your choice of donor.

14

Talking about Donor Conception

> [There is] *clear authority within both our legal and social community that identity is the crucial part of the right to know. Any move by a parent or State to try to conceal, destroy or prevent a child from knowing his or her origins—both biological and social—is to be correctly regarded a human rights violation.'*
>
> **His Honour Chief Judge John Pascoe**[192]

> *My parents were told it was just like giving blood and no big deal. And never to tell me. It makes me angry that some of that is still going on today almost forty years later! Clinics definitely know better now, they just care more about profits than people.*
>
> **Australian donor-conceived adult (NSW)**

In the past, parents of adopted children were counselled *not* to tell their children that they were adopted. The same advice was given to parents of donor-conceived children as is stated in this passage quoting the opinion of Dr Philip Bloom:

> *For the child's sake particularly I prefer that absolutely nobody but the parents themselves and myself should know of the insemination therapy. My last advice to the parents is that under no circumstances should they, or need they, ever tell the child the method of conception—in fact they should forget about it themselves.*[193]

Now we know better.[194]

All people have a right to know their genetic origins,[195] and research tells us that many donor-conceived people feel strongly about their right to access genetic information.[196] Talking to your child about their conception is a profoundly personal experience and may be associated with a multitude of feelings, including fear and anxiety. It is not a simple one-off event, but a series of ongoing discussions as your child develops their identity, language and cognitive ability. The practice of initiating conversations that evolve over time (none of which require perfection) also lets your child know that a perpetually safe space exists in which to discuss the topic of donor conception and that no one feels uncomfortable about how they came into being.

Why don't people tell?

> *We used an egg donor and my wife refuses to tell our child. Both of our families know. I told her that our child deserves to know the truth, and that I am happy to tell our child. She said she'd kick me out of the house if I even bring up the subject again. My wife's family who we live with, also does not want the family secret disclosed to our child.*
>
> **Australian recipient parent**

Despite current recommendations for disclosure, many people are not telling their children they are donor-conceived. In some cases, parents withhold this information with good intentions, but without really understanding the long-term ramifications of doing so. Sometimes, in cases where double donation has been used, a parent might tell their children they were conceived using a sperm donor, but neglect to mention the egg donor. Finding out later in life that you are not genetically related to a parent is often referred to as 'Non-Parent Expected' (NPE) or a Misattributed Parentage Event (MPE). Support groups exist to help people in this situation.

What are some of the reasons people don't tell? Some of them are discussed under the following headings.

Shame and infertility

> *To know who you are and where you came from is not a privilege, it is a right. It is something ingrained in us from the very beginning. To have to change those beliefs later is damaging. It breaks ones being. Everyone should know their truth. No one should be a secret or a burden. One should be able to express the truth of who they are and not feel ashamed or clandestine.*
>
> **Kate Richards (Australian donor-conceived adult [Vic.])**

Infertility affects many people and frequently manifests as shame for the sufferer. When these painful feelings are carried in silence and remain unacknowledged, the result can manifest as a decision not to tell. Sometimes people also choose to guard the infertility secrets of their partners.

If you or your partner feel shame about your infertility, it is important to acknowledge these feelings and explore the source of your concerns. There are many resources available to assist you in the form of articles, books, support groups and professionally trained grief counsellors. Healing from past hurts and personal trauma can be a long and challenging road, but it is vital you do not pass on your shame to your child for whom it may present as shame of being donor-conceived.

Beliefs and discrimination

> *My parents told their parents and siblings. No one else knew. My grandparents, aunts, and uncles never said anything to me about it. I wasn't permitted to tell anyone about being donor-conceived. I wish my parents would have allowed me to be out to anyone and everyone. Making me believe that only certain people could know about it made it very apparent that there was a lot of shame for them surrounding who I am and where I came from.*
>
> **American donor-conceived adult**

Religious, cultural, ethnic and psychosocial constraints may impact a person's decision to tell their child about their origins. Some groups are opposed to the use of donated gametes and, often, different opinions and levels of acceptance are observed within the same group. For LGBTQIA+ families, simply standing up for your rights to create a family that does not align with heteronormative expectations may feel onerous and demanding. A lifetime of values, beliefs and worship, and pressure or disapproval from family members, can be extremely influential in a person's decision-making process in regard to keeping their child's conception story a secret. In some cultures, genetics play an extremely important role in families and connection to biological family and ancestors is significant. In these circumstances, a person might feel shame about not being genetically connected to their child and that can impact their decision not to tell.

It's important to know that you don't need to tell *everyone* about your child's conception story, particularly if you think it may cause harm to your child and your family (see the following section about 'Protecting your child'). Telling your child, on the other hand, is crucial.

Protecting your child

> *I was told at thirty-three. My mother always wanted to tell me, but she worried I'd be bullied or feel alone. By the time the internet and online support groups came along I was in my teens and twenties and dealing with mental health issues, which she didn't want to add to by disclosing. Then she waited a few extra years because she was so scared of how I'd react that she couldn't quite work up the courage. I wish I'd known earlier, but I understand that she was trying to do the right thing for me.*
>
> **Australian donor-conceived adult (NSW)**

Sometimes parents feel they should protect their child's privacy by keeping the details of their conception from others, leaving it for the child to later determine whether the story is one they may, or may not, wish to share. As an extension of this, some parents fear their child may be bullied by others if their genetic origins are known, or that they might be seen as 'different'. While this may be legitimate in rare circumstances, it is still vital your child knows their origins (see 'How and when to tell' later in this chapter).

Fear of not being genetically related and fear of loss

> *I was worried it would upset my parents when I started talking to them about how I wanted to reach out to my bio father and I was super conscious of being sensitive to them but, in fact, being able to have those conversations with them has only made our relationship stronger. They've even met my bio father now and my Dad talks about how it's been a positive thing for him. I think I struck it lucky to have parents who have been so loving and supportive.*
>
> **Australian donor-conceived adult (Vic.)**

If a person has not worked through their grief about being the non-biological parent, it can affect their ability to bond with a child and have long-term impacts. The good news is that, when feelings have been worked through and a parent-child relationship has been built on trust, a healthy parent–child attachment does *not* depend on genetic links and can develop over time through consistent care and emotional sharing.[197]

> *I see a ton of parents being very wound up with concerns that contact with a biological parent* [donor] *will be harmful or confusing. I've never met a donor-conceived person who is confused about their parentage and I definitely feel clear on mine. It's only the adults who struggle in this situation.*
>
> **American donor-conceived adult**

If you fear your child will no longer love you when they meet the donor, this appears to have little foundation. When donor-conceived people tell us about finding the donor, they generally tell us it had absolutely no impact on how much they love their raising parents. A 2019 Australian study reviewing retrospective access to previously anonymous Victorian sperm donors' records found a common theme in the applicants' statements regarding the process and their experience of identifying and meeting their biological parent (sperm donor). None of the donor-conceived people spoke negatively about their raising parents and several went so far as to reassure their biological parent that they were not looking for a replacement father or a father figure.[198]

It's important to recognise that if you feel a loss from not being genetically connected to your child, at some stage your child may also feel the same way about not being connected to their biological parent (the donor).

Never finding the 'right time'

> *I have so much empathy for my mother and I feel so awful for her that she had to carry this secret for so long. This situation really hurts everyone.*
>
> **Australian donor-conceived adult (NSW)**

Sometimes people have every intention of telling their children their conception stories, but never find the right words or the right time to do so. This generally creates a sense of ongoing anxiety in the parents, the discomfort building with time.

Ongoing denial

> *When I discovered in my forties that I was donor conceived, my parents initially wanted it kept secret. But this isn't just about them, it's about me, it's about the family I'm building and potentially the genetic links I have in my own community. I brought them around to being open about it with time, but I can't imagine having kept silent long term, or how hard it would be for a child.*
>
> **Terry Masson (Australian donor-conceived adult [SA])**

In situations where parents are in complete denial regarding their child's conception story, a donor-conceived person who discovers the truth about their origins may even be asked by a parent to maintain the secret they have held onto for such a long time. In rare cases, a parent may continue to deny the details of their child's conception, even when confronted with the evidence.

All of the responses presented on the previous pages are genuine and require self-reflection and abundant amounts of self-compassion. Know that if you, or your partner, are experiencing hesitation in telling your child their conception story, you are not alone.

So, what can you do?

First, before commencing the process of donor conception, give yourself all the time you need to work through your concerns until you arrive at a place of feeling comfortable about talking to your future child. Seek help if necessary. According to psychotherapist and fertility counsellor Jana Rupnow, this will: allow you to fully embrace the telling process; contribute to your child's healthy identity development; and enhance your parent–child relationship through a foundation built on honesty and trust.[199]

If you already have a donor-conceived child and have not yet told them their conception story, there are numerous tools and resources available to assist you to do so (see 'How and when to tell' later in this chapter).

How are secrets uncovered?

> *I personally always felt a bit like the cuckoo in the nest; didn't quite fit.*
>
> **Australian donor-conceived adult (NSW)**

It's really hard to keep a secret forever, especially one of such huge magnitude. Certainly, it might seem like an easy thing to do when your child is young, but is likely to become more difficult as your child gets older. Either way, keeping the details of your child's conception a secret is a hazardous affair and requires sustained and relentless focus to avoid tripping up.

Many donor-conceived people (particularly those who were previously unaware of their conception story) speak of feeling that something was a little 'off'; an indefinable absence of something in their lives; an incomplete identity; or that they do not resemble their parents or other family members in any way. Some even describe a strange void in which they recognised that their own intelligence far surpassed that of their parents (possibly because many recipient parents choose highly intelligent donors). For some it can lead them to speculate about whether a parent has had an affair, or whether they were adopted.

So how do people find out the truth?

> *I'm a late discovery donor-conceived person. I discovered the truth in a family argument (as an adult) which made the whole disclosure even more painful.*
>
> **Hayley King (British donor-conceived adult and recipient parent)**

For those that aren't told by their parents, many discover the details of their conception by completing a DNA test. In some cases, people discover they are donor-conceived when a sibling has completed a DNA test and makes contact. Some people find out when they develop a health condition that involves reviewing their genetic history. Others realise (in some cases, during a high school project) that their blood type is simply not possible based on their parents' genetics. In rare cases, a person might discover their origins when a family member requires an organ donation. Even more distressing perhaps, some donor-conceived people find out when family separation occurs and a family member, in a moment of anger and release of suppressed emotions, spills the beans about their relationship to their child. Alternatively, there may also be an accidental or deliberate disclosure by a family member or friend.

The cost of secrecy

> *Lying to your children is an excellent way to destroy your relationship with them. I know several donor-conceived people who discovered the truth via a DNA test and no longer speak to their parents.*
>
> **Erin Jackson (founder of We Are Donor Conceived)**

It is true that some donor-conceived people are simply surprised by a secret unveiled and do not express any ill-feelings towards their raising parents for keeping their conception 'hush-hush', embracing the news with pleasure and wonder; a new world of family trees to explore and discover. Some describe the discovery as a mere blip in the journey of life.

However, in many cases, the revelation of such a secret can bring with it shock, anger, grief, resentment, confusion about identity, mistrust and, in some cases, estrangement. A simple lie, spanning years (and, in many cases, decades) ruptures dramatically, the deluge winding its way far beyond the four walls of a once-happy home, extending downstream to other families onto newly-discovered siblings; their parents; friends; the donor-conceived person's own children. The lie must be addressed, broken down into its fundamental components and laid bare; the when, why and how of it all a harrowing business to work through after years of secrecy.

Bearing the burden of others' secrets

> *I actually have a bit of a pickle about this secrecy thing. Because I do have quite a bit of contact with a donor-conceived sister, but her kids can't know, because her mother can't know that she knows, and the kids would tell grandma. So they don't know that I'm their aunt, I'm just 'Angela' to them. Which will mean that my kid probably can't know. But I'm not really sure that I'm willing to lie to the kid. Sooooooo . . . do you just chuck an important relationship over bullshit secrecy? I mean, of course not. But the whole thing is so complicated.*
>
> **American donor-conceived adult and recipient parent**

Some donor-conceived people don't care either way about their genetic connections, but many feel the burden of other people's secrets; their shame. For some it is an enduring message that repeatedly expresses the sentiment that they must pretend not to exist and, instead, must hide in the shadows of a dark secret that ought to stay buried.

A conception secret can have far-reaching consequences. There are many victims but, generally, this plight falls upon the donor-conceived person.

For instance, sometimes a donor-conceived person is placed in the awkward position of setting up a time to 'have a talk with the parents' to let them know they've become aware they were donor-conceived. Alternatively, in order to avoid hurting them, the donor-conceived adult might decide not to tell their parents they have discovered their donor-conceived status.

When it comes to donor-conceived siblings, a donor-conceived person might discover via direct-to-consumer DNA testing that they have multiple siblings, all (or many) of whom have known each other from a young age, and they are now forced to navigate their way into their sibling group as an adult, having missed out on years (or, in some cases, decades) of connection. Alternatively, a donor-conceived person could be contacted by a sibling who, having completed a DNA test, is curious about their possible relationship. They are then placed in the uncomfortable position of deciding whether it is their responsibility to tell their sibling that they too are donor-conceived, or, alternatively, that their parent donated gametes many years ago.

Sometimes a donor-conceived person is unclear about boundaries and whether to contact their biological parent or siblings on birthdays and other celebratory days. Occasionally donor-conceived people are refused attendance at the funeral of a sibling or biological parent because they are not considered family, or to avoid the possibility of people asking how they know the deceased and revealing a long-held family secret.

Some donor-conceived people experience anxiety, depression and, on occasions, post-traumatic stress disorder after discovering their entire identity is based on lies.

Other risks of secrecy

In addition to the shock potentially experienced by a donor-conceived person who discovers their true conception story, there are also other more sobering and disastrous possibilities that can arise from this single act of secrecy. Some of these are discussed under the following headings.

Medical conditions

> *I believe I have found my donor, although we have only chatted by email, and the record keepers refusing to confirm if it's him or not despite both our consents being given. Without any connection to his family (at his request), I have no knowledge of anything new that may crop up, and a limited/anecdotal family history. What worries me more is how will I know when he passes? Will it just be six months of radio silence and then I give up?*
>
> **Terry Masson (Australian donor-conceived adult [SA])**

When a person's conception is kept a secret, there is generally an assumption made about parentage. For example, a donor-conceived person with heterosexual parents is likely to assume that their raising father is also their genetic father. This may have an impact in one of two ways: If the donor-conceived person's raising father presents with an inherited disease or genetic condition, the child or adult may live in fear of experiencing that condition themselves. Alternatively, if the donor presents with a genetic condition, the donor-conceived child will have no awareness of this or of the need to seek preventative measures.

While not all diseases and disorders can be tested for, knowing what we *might* inherit can help us prevent, or prepare for, situations that may affect our health and cause illness. Knowing medical aspects of our genetic makeup ensures that we provide correct information to health professionals—which could be lifesaving.

Consanguinity

Consanguinity means 'descending from the same ancestor' or 'being related by blood'. A person who doesn't know they are donor-conceived could unwittingly form a relationship with a person to whom they are related. See Chapter 9, 'Choosing Your Donor[s]'.

Genetic sexual attraction

Donor-conceived people are potentially at risk of the attraction which can arise towards siblings (and cousins and parents) when they first meet or are reunited as adults. See Chapter 9, 'Choosing Your Donor[s]' where this is discussed in more detail.

Direct-to-consumer DNA testing

Direct-to-consumer DNA testing has made testing for genetic links accessible to everyone, making it possible to locate genetic relatives previously unknown. See Chapter 15, 'Donor and Sibling Linking'.

Telling

> *I'm personally fine with the way I was conceived, and I was never deceived. However, I just want to throw out there that you can be honest with your child about being donor-conceived and still do harm in the way you talk about it. If your child feels like it's hush hush, if they feel guilty for their curiosity, there's still an issue.*
>
> **American donor-conceived adult**

Research indicates it is best to tell our children their conception story early, so they never remember a time when they didn't know.[200] Pursuant to this knowledge, Australian clinics are required to outline the benefits of early disclosure to intended parents.[201] Adoptees who learned of their status at three years or older reported more distress and decreased life satisfaction than those told before they turned three years of age.[202] We know that many donor-conceived people express feelings and emotions about their conception story that parallel those experienced by adoptees, but does the data show any similarities between the two situations?

One longitudinal study of eighty-seven donor-conceived families concluded that the earlier the donor-conceived children were told their conception story, the better the quality of family relationships and adolescent psychological wellbeing.[203] In other words, telling your child their conception story early does appear to have positive consequences. For instance, communicating honestly and openly builds a foundation of trust between you and your child and, subsequently, has a positive impact on your child's relationships with others. Trust also contributes to secure parent–child attachments which, in turn, can positively influence future relationships. As your child's adolescence looms and identity creation is at its peak, having forged a solid foundation of trust can assist you in helping your child develop their identity with all of the information available and will allow them to work through how being donor-conceived fits with their sense of self.[204]

Parents can also benefit from telling children their conception story early. The same longitudinal study referred to above indicated that, when children learned about their conception details before the age of seven, their mothers showed lower levels of anxiety and depression.[205]

Telling early allows parents to have a few practice runs, to get the story 'right' in a way that works well and is comfortable for them. Parents have no need to spend sleepless nights waiting for that perfect moment and there are no tense discussions about whether to tell the child on their seventh birthday, eleventh Christmas, or before they start high school. The child has just always known—even before they could understand—and being donor-conceived forms a natural part of their identity and their place in the world.

There is no 'telling event'.

As your child gets older and comes to understand more about how they came to exist, the conversation can continue at an age-appropriate pace, with consideration given to the types of questions asked, the cognisance displayed and the emotions subtly (or overtly) influencing those enquiries. Whether your child will feel comfortable sharing their feelings and asking questions will depend on a range of factors, including: your own levels of awareness, comfort and communication about the conception story; your child's level of self-awareness and emotional intelligence; and their personality.[206] And just because they're not asking questions, don't assume they don't have any.

Some parents feel hesitant about disclosing the existence of half-siblings to their child, but consider the risk of your child being angry with you later when they find out they have multiple siblings and have missed out on years of getting to know them. What meaning will your child place on your decision not to disclose this information about their genetic relatives? We tell our children about cousins, aunties, uncles, and so on; we meet up with them; we share celebrations—so why not mention siblings?

As a parent, initiating conversations like this when our children are young enables them to construct their own life story with all of the pieces available. It allows them to weave the pieces into the puzzle as they see fit—discovering and developing connections, and making decisions about who they wish to have in their life, and who they do not. Then, once your child is old enough to be fully cognisant of the situation, it is no longer your story to tell and your child can take the lead—with your continuing support and guidance.

If you haven't told your child their conception story yet, there's no time like the present. If you feel you need help to get the conversation started, particularly if your child is entering their teens, there's plenty of assistance available. (See 'Useful tools and resources' at the back of this book for links to online sources containing additional resources, blog articles and the latest updates about donor conception.)

How and when to tell

Finding the right time and, especially, the right words to tell your child they are donor-conceived can be daunting. If this describes you, the great news is that there is a multitude of children's books available to do the work for you—in the early years at least. Some books are better than others, so it's worth doing your research to understand what it is you actually want to tell your child and which books do that. For instance, a book might perpetuate a harmful industry narrative like 'the donor is just providing a cell'; or reinforce heteronormative family structures only, when you want to educate your child about diversity. Many people make their own children's books, or edit existing published books to include the personal details they know about their donor to help enrich their child's story. A photo book containing images of the various aspects of your child's conception can also be a valuable resource and will help to convey the message that you are proud and happy about your unique family.

It's also important to be mindful that being donor-conceived is only one aspect of your child's life and, as one donor-conceived person said to me:

> *Books are great, but don't shove it down their throats and read it every night because that's just weird—unless, of course, your child requests the same book every night. . .*

So, once you've taken the first steps towards telling your child, you may find your confidence grows and that the conversation evolves as your child starts to ask more questions or you want to convey more detail. Alternatively, sometimes your child may wish to speak to someone else about their conception story, so it may be of value to suggest a supportive family member, friend or even a counsellor trained in the nuances of donor conception.

One of the other things to consider is that children can generally grasp more complex scenarios than we give them credit for. For example, one common and heteronormative industry message is that children will be confused by a non-traditional family structure or by having more than two parents. But children generally understand quite clearly when they have two mothers, or two fathers, or a parent and a step-parent, or that they live with their grandparents so, they'll usually get it if you want to tell them they've got three (or four) parents (one of whom doesn't live with them), three sets of grandparents, two siblings that live with them and fifteen that don't. It's adults that over-complicate things, so try not to project your fears and misgivings onto your children. Just tell them the facts, using age-appropriate language, and move on. And if they don't quite comprehend it all right away, they will later, so it's important to use the correct descriptions from the outset and avoid the need for conversations like, 'Hey, sweetheart, you know how you've been calling him Uncle Pete . . .'

Another aspect to consider is the manner in which you impart information directly to your child or, alternatively, when you are conversing with others while your child is listening. Are you speaking with confidence and love about the way in which you created your family? Are you normalising your child's conception by using language and tone that embraces their uniqueness to you as their parent, while simultaneously embracing the diversity of family structures? Are you leaving the door open for questions to be asked later, or are you conveying the message that all further conversation has now been terminated?

Pregnancy and infancy

Babies in utero can start to hear low-pitched sounds from about sixteen weeks and can hear more high-pitched sounds later in the pregnancy. They can certainly hear their gestational parent's voice. Some people read to their baby while they are in utero and there is no reason why you and your partner can't start talking to your child about their conception story *before* they are born. Once they've arrived, you can talk to them while feeding, rocking them to sleep, going for a walk; there are many opportunities to practice the wording of your story and, in the early days of infancy when your child can't talk back, the 'conversation' will be one-way and very easy.

Toddlers, pre-school and early primary school

Young children between the ages of three and five usually only need simple information and have a short attention span so, again, just stick to the basic facts. Children at this age are very literal and love to hear stories about themselves, so you will have very few challenges regarding their conception story. Ensure your tone is always positive because your child will take their cues from you.[207]

Cory Silverberg's book, *What Makes a Baby,*[208] is useful for explaining gametes and the act of conception in an uncomplicated gender-neutral manner, using simple statements to describe how a baby is made from an egg and a sperm, each of which contains unique stories that mix to become one story, and that a baby needs a uterus in which to grow.

You can also explain that families come in various shapes and sizes and provide different examples, such as two mums, two dads, a single parent, three parents who don't all live together or four that do, and so on. If you feel comfortable doing so, you may wish to lend your child's teacher a book so it can be read to the whole class, discussed as a group and questions from the children can be answered. This may help your child feel supported, as well as put boundaries in place for further discussion, if necessary. Often children just need to know 'what is' and then they will move on.

Primary school children

> *I was told when I was seven. By then my concept of self and where I fit within my family was already established. This is a significant and unnecessary emotional burden to place on a child when the concept of being donor-conceived could be woven into identity formation from the beginning.*
>
> **Australian donor-conceived adult (Qld)**

As children's cognitive development progresses, they can understand more complex information and you can begin to expand on topics related to conception and reproduction. One of the things we know now is that using the correct anatomical terms for body parts helps children in several distinct ways. The use of correct language, rather than euphemisms such as 'privates' or 'undercarriage', prevents shame or embarrassment being unintentionally attached to those parts of the body. It also generates a safe space for ongoing conversations to be had with children about their bodies and about sexuality and gender.

An exception to this is cases when referring to anatomically correct terms might contribute to gender dysphoria (anxiety and depression related to conflict between a person's sex assigned at birth and the gender with which they identify).

In terms of donor conception, using correct terminology creates the possibility for open dialogue in order to discuss, very early in a child's life, how they were conceived. This might involve explaining the circumstances of their conception in a little more detail, including that you required help from another person to create them.

Children of primary school age may also start to develop a little more interest in their conception story and the part it plays in the formation of their identity as they are exposed to more external influences such as television, or other children and their respective family structures.[209]

Children will also start to form opinions and beliefs about their conception story based on your feelings and what you are saying, but your non-verbal communication will have the biggest impact. For instance, if you have unresolved negativity or shame, you will convey that unconsciously.

If you do not talk about your child's conception with them at all, you are actually telling them a great deal.[210] Initiate conversations, give your child your full attention and answer their questions to the best of your ability.[211]

Young children can express an interest in genetics and demonstrate curiosity related to which aspects of themselves they've inherited from their biological parents. If you are a non-biological parent, you can also discuss distinguishing behaviours and aspects of yourself that have influenced your child through nurture. This is also a good time to discuss that, while genetics are important, families are also created with love. Your child might also be interested in the details of the fertility treatment you underwent to create them.[212]

If you feel comfortable, at the start of each school year (with your child's permission) it could be helpful to inform the new teacher about your child's donor-conceived status and ensure they will be supportive should a need arise. You might explain that your child may, or may not, wish to talk with the other children about being donor-conceived and highlight any potential issues that could arise. For example, if your child says they have dozens of siblings, they may be accused of lying. Or they may be constantly questioned about why they don't have a dad (or other parent). You can then work with the teacher to discuss how you would like these potential scenarios to be managed.

There are multiple books available for this age group, including some that involve fictional stories featuring donor-conceived children in a variety of family structures. This may help to create an awareness in your child that there are plenty of other donor-conceived children out there and that there is nothing 'different' about them.

Tweens and teens

> *I cried when they told me at age nine. I was very concerned with my appearance because I look so different than my mother. Anytime I expressed concern that I was too tall or I hated my hair color, that should have been a clue. But they also never asked what I wanted. And if I'd been asked, I would have told them I wanted to know my biological father as a child.*
>
> **American donor-conceived adult**

As children develop more independence and experience the physical, emotional and mental changes that come with puberty, they may become more self-conscious and embarrassed about discussing such topics as reproduction and conception.[213] Identity creation also expands to a critical undertaking as adolescents search for a sense of self and explore their personal values, beliefs and goals.[214] Jana Rupnow explains: 'The question, "Who am I?" becomes central to a teenager's development'.[215]

A small 2016 study involving twenty-three donor-conceived adolescents found that curiosity about connecting with their siblings was focused mainly on what information they could glean about the *donor* and, as an extension of that, about *themselves*. The findings also suggested that the ID Release policy of eighteen years of age is several years too late.[216]

If you have been talking to your child about their conception from a young age, you may find they now start 'owning' their story and become selective about the people with whom they share this personal information. As a parent, you may find that you need their permission to discuss their conception with others. Teenagers generally do not wish to be seen as a curiosity or different from others in any way. Sometimes donor-conceived children who are raised by LGBTQIA+

parents may not wish to share this fact with others because of fears related to discrimination, homophobia or transphobia. Others may feel uncomfortable about describing the sexual and reproductive terminology required to explain their conception.[217] In all cases, it's important to respect and support your child's choices about what they do with this information.

If you are telling your child about their conception for the first time as a tween or teenager, they may experience strong emotions including shock, anger, mistrust and anxiety. They may also experience sadness about not sharing a genetic connection with family and encounter challenges coping with the reactions when they share the news with friends.[218] Prior to sharing the information about their conception with your child, it may be worth seeking assistance from a counsellor, another donor-conceived person or a supportive friend or family member. You may also find that your child does not wish to talk to you about it, so finding another person with whom they feel comfortable sharing their feelings can be helpful.

If you have information about your child's donor, you may wish to print it and leave it in your child's room for them to look through when they're ready. Research involving donor-conceived teenagers indicates they feel they have a right to know their conception story, that they prefer their parents to do the telling and that parents should offer an explanation about why they had not previously told them.[219]

Arguably, one of the most important things to do is to listen to your child. Listen to their questions, their anger, shock (or any other emotions they might express), and provide the reasons why you withheld the truth. But do not, under any circumstances, place the burden on your child of your own shame, regret, sadness or fear. An extremely common theme described by donor-conceived people is the emotional labour they go through to protect their parents from hurt. Remember, your child is not responsible for your feelings. If you need further assistance unpacking any fallout from the conversation with your child, seek assistance elsewhere from a partner, a friend or a counsellor.

Adults

> *I found out I was donor-conceived at age thirty-eight. It felt like the ground fell out from underneath me. I cried for three months and I had a 'good' outcome. I found my siblings and my donor who have been happy to meet. Two years on, and I still have days where I feel immense sadness at the time lost with my siblings, the lies told to me for thirty-eight years and the loss of biological connection to my father.*
>
> **Australian donor-conceived adult (ACT)**

Adults are more likely to have negative reactions to finding out they are donor-conceived[220] and, regardless of their response, they will need time to process the information. Adults might feel they need to completely redefine their identity and the way they have positioned themselves in their family. Some donor-conceived people describe how this new knowledge taints all of their childhood memories. It is likely to be helpful for them to talk to other donor-conceived people or a counsellor.

There's no question that telling adult children is challenging and, in some cases, has caused harm to families in cases where parents were advised at the time of conception not to tell.[221] So, in order to prepare yourself, it may be helpful to seek assistance prior to having the conversation and, again, to ensure you do not burden your child with your own feelings.

Late disclosure: Tips for telling

Following are some suggestions you might wish to consider when telling your child (as an older child or adult) that they are donor-conceived.

- Rather than a public place, choose a familiar location which offers privacy, such as your home.
- Choose a time when everyone involved in the conversation isn't busy, so there is plenty of time for discussion.
- Avoid telling directly after a relationship breakdown.

- Do *not* tell your child on their birthday or other significant celebration day, in case the telling creates an unpleasant anniversary for them.
- If you have more than one child, tell them together (unless one child is not donor-conceived; in which case tell that child immediately *after* the donor-conceived child has been told).
- Tell as a couple (if that applies), even if you are separated (and if it is possible and safe to do so).
- Prepare by considering what you would like to say and rehearsing it, if that helps.
- If you are better at the written word, write a letter—but be present to discuss it when it is read.[222]
- Apologise for keeping the secret from them and for not telling them sooner.
- Use clear and concise factual information.
- Try to control your emotions and centre the conversation on your child, *not* on yourself. Don't make them feel they need to comfort you.
- Do *not* tell them how wanted they were, or talk in-depth about how difficult it was for you to conceive them (see 'Upsetting phrases and comments' later in this chapter).
- Let them know that they can tell, or not tell, anyone they want to about this new information.
- Listen—really listen—and, if they don't want to talk, accept that.
- Let them know they may have donor-conceived siblings.
- Minimise the resulting emotional labour for your child by providing them with as much information as you have about the donor (but understand they may need time first to process finding out they are donor-conceived). When the time is right provide personal details, photos, etc. relating to the donor, as well as information about the clinic so they can seek out their siblings if they wish. Do as much of the groundwork as you can yourself because, sometimes, clinics and banks refuse to provide this kind of information to donor-conceived people.

- Let them know how they can connect with other donor-conceived people to support them with processing this new information (see Chapter 15, 'Donor and sibling linking').
- If they are open to it, arrange for some counselling. Pay for the counselling yourself. Consider engaging in some counselling as a whole family.
- Depending on their age, you may like to offer them the option of a direct-to-consumer DNA test kit. Pay for the DNA test yourself.
- Check in with your donor-conceived child soon after and in the weeks following the discussion. While they might not have (or might not display) an immediate reaction to the news at the time of its telling, this could change quickly. Give them space if they need it, but keep checking in over the weeks, months and years.

Telling family and members of your support network

> *You will need to decide as your child grows up who needs to know, but a general climate of openness within the family, where a child gets the message that this is a safe topic to talk about, is helpful.*
>
> **Olivia Montuschi**
> **(Cofounder of the Donor Conception Network, UK)**

Regardless of your relationship status, it's important to have supportive people around you when you become a parent. Telling friends, family and colleagues about your child's conception story may build the foundations for healthy conversations and ongoing support.

Sometimes people aren't sure about who they should tell and who they shouldn't. For this reason, it's important to identify the difference between privacy and secrecy. Jana Rupnow defines 'privacy' as the withholding of information from public view and from those people who don't need to know, whereas 'secrecy' involves withholding information from everyone, including those who should know.[223] In other words, depending on your circumstances, you do not need to divulge the information about your child's birth to absolutely everyone, but it's vital you tell your child—and the number of people you tell may expand over time.

It's important to ensure you do not place your child in the position of having to maintain a secret that you have initiated and perpetuated. Learning to set boundaries may take some practice, particularly when people express disapproval of your plans or ask inappropriate and offensive questions. Over time, when questions are asked in front of your child, you can learn to respond in healthy ways that honour their story.

Having a conversation with your child about the difference between 'secrecy' and 'privacy' is also very important so they understand that, while being donor-conceived is not a secret, they can still choose who they tell. Sometimes children become tired of or bored with explaining their conception story, so you may be able to assist them with suggestions of healthy responses or provide them with scripted answers that deflect the questions.

So how do you know who to tell? A good question to ask yourself is, 'Is telling this person in the best interests of my child?' For instance, is it better to withhold information from family members and friends whom you suspect will disapprove or judge, only for your child to discover later that these people are unaware of their conception story? Will your child translate that into shame of being donor-conceived, or will you be able to provide a reasonable explanation about why particular people don't know? Alternatively, can you inform the potential disapprovers, let them bear the burden of their own discomfort and leave your child free to own their donor-conceived status? Of course, where there is a risk of physical, mental or emotional harm involved with certain people (including relatives), the decision to hold your story close may be easy. For instance, some donor-conceived people report being rejected by family, being made unwelcome at family gatherings and being left out of grandparents' wills. In some cases, people have even been left out of their non-biological raising parent's will.

The way in which you strategise disclosure to others can be challenging. Consider what you know and do what you feel will provide the best outcomes for your child. Remember, your child is watching and will learn how to respond based on your responses and actions.

Another thing to consider is that, if your family is built on secrets and no one knows you've used a donor, might that kind of secrecy also extend to your brother who's told no one he's become a sperm donor? In which case, would you recognise your brother's profile when selecting a donor or would you, instead, be attracted to it because of the similarities to you and your family? I'll leave that with you . . .

Responding to strangers

> *I don't think conception details are any business of the random people in shops, waiting rooms, at the bus stop. But if your verbal toddler says something, go with the flow and don't hush them.*
>
> **Australian recipient parent**

Then there are the strangers . . .

What happens when someone you don't know very well or a perfect stranger asks about your child's conception? Enquiries like, 'Where's Daddy?', 'Who is the birth mother?' and 'How much does fertility treatment cost?' can be confronting and intrusive. Your response could depend on how you feel at that moment and the level of respect shown to you by the questioner. And you don't have to answer. You don't have to explain to every person all of the time and it is likely that, over time, you will develop confidence with managing these types of questions. Nevertheless, it's still important to consider that, if you choose to avoid a direct question, lie, or tell an 'alternative' story in front of your child, your child may wonder why their conception story is cause for concealment.

Feelings evolve

> *How people feel about being donor-conceived can change over time. All reactions and responses are a possibility and aren't a reflection on parenting, or how well-adjusted or 'happy' someone is.*
>
> **Australian donor-conceived adult (NSW)**

How people feel about being donor-conceived varies significantly, regardless of whether you told them from Day 1, or when they were a teenager. All responses are normal and it's important to know that, even if your child appears to withdraw from you, they still need your support. You are the anchor they can return to.[224] Like most things in life, emotions and feelings evolve over time. What's not on the radar one day, may appear front and centre the next. Many donor-conceived people have little or no interest in their conception story for years, until one day something happens: they are contacted by a sibling, complete a DNA test, have their own child, become unwell, and so on. How we feel about certain aspects of our lives can be fluid.

Again, some donor-conceived people don't place great importance on their genetic connections, but the ones who do tell us of their need to be provided with the space to work through the process of their conception, permission to explore who they are and the freedom to develop their own sense of self.

> *I'm a queer recipient parent and I am also donor-conceived. I didn't learn I was donor-conceived until I was trying to get pregnant. I have had to hide my grief and longing for fear of hurting my parents. It sucks! I've recently connected with my donor and it has been so wonderful. People always say 'Oh . . . how are your parents dealing with that?!' Like I have to carry the weight of my parents' feelings about this? Ugh! It's so complicated. I always want to honor my kids' feelings about being donor-conceived, and they do not have to hide their feelings to protect mine.*
>
> **American donor-conceived adult**

Likewise, if they are feeling sad about their conception story, or any aspect of it, don't try to make them happy. If they're feeling angry, let them be angry. Don't try to fix it. Give them permission to express their emotions and provide them with healthy ways to do it. Seek help if you don't know how.

As Jana Rupnow suggests, perhaps the most important thing you can do is just listen and tell them you understand. The consequences of not allowing our children to experience their feelings is that we teach them to suppress their feelings; we also send the message that they are only allowed to be positive about their conception story.[225]

Further potential outcomes are that your teenage/adult child may seek emotional support and guidance from another source (often via donor-conceived support groups) without your knowledge, exploring their genetics covertly. Some donor-conceived people even wait until their raising parents have died before they investigate.

Language and terminology

> *I don't have a donor. My parents had a donor. Choosing to ignore and misname the literal relationship is distancing and is solely for the parent's benefit, not the child's. Now, as an adult, I have seven parents; a biological mother who I call Mum, a step-mother who I call Sarah, a mother-in-law who I call Judy, the man who raised me who I call Dad, a biological father who I call Jim, a step-father who I call Peter, and a father-in-law who I call Sam. Lucky me to have so many parental figures! And all quite easily differentiated in my view.*
>
> **Australian donor-conceived adult (WA)**

Language is constantly shifting and evolving, meandering along its own unique and distinctive path, changing from one generation to the next. This is definitely true in the world of donor conception. Language also plays an important part in the LGBTQIA+ community and heteronormative terms such as 'mother' and 'father' can often reinforce the notion that families without these two figures are not 'normal' or legitimate.

So, how do we, as parents, manage all of the terminology; the contexts; the scenarios? Should your child's needs be a consideration when it comes to the language used, even when you're not so comfortable or pleased with it? What if you advocate for something—even if it's come from a donor-conceived adult—but your donor-conceived child tells you they don't like it?

Ultimately, if we want our children to embrace their unique identities, they need to be given the green light to make their own decisions regarding the terms they wish to use, even if these don't align with our own wants and needs, or the advice we have been given by a counsellor.

Factors to consider when discussing donor conception

Refer to your donor with respect

> *I think it's tied in with the genetic bewilderment many donor-conceived people experience. If half of you is erased, what does that do to your sense of self and identity? If the raising parents send a message that the person who is half of you does not matter and his/her/they are 'only a cell', 'just like blood donation'—how can that not have dehumanising effects?*
>
> **Katie (Australian former egg donor)**

Donor conception is a sensitive subject for many and, while the assortment of labels and pet names for various parties (and physical instruments) involved in the process can be bandied about with fun intent, sometimes those monikers offend. As with any sensitive situation, or out of plain old respect, it is important to use language and tone that show consideration for others.

For instance, should you joke about your donor? Are the details of your child's conception an amusing story to relate at a barbecue on a sunny afternoon, or at a dinner party after the third bottle of Shiraz—the tale about 'the bloke who jizzed in a jar', or 'the chick who laid a whole lot of high-quality eggs'? While jokes can be funny, they can also be extremely offensive to your donor who may have had genuine altruistic intent to help you start a family. They can also be especially concerning to your child—a human being who needs to know their existence is not the result of an amusing skit.

Regardless of your feelings about the donor you select, it's important to remember they will contribute half of your child's genetic makeup and will subsequently have an impact on your child's creation of identity.

Provide accurate details

> *As a donor-conceived person my advice would be to avoid any descriptions that could lead your child to start fantasising about a kind and generous person when the reality may well be very different. Not saying there are no mature altruistic donors, but let's not idealise the situation or attribute qualities that aren't there.*
>
> **Australian donor-conceived adult (NSW)**

Another factor to be mindful of is the *manner* in which you describe your donor(s). For instance, many people describe the donor as 'a nice man', 'a kind woman', 'a generous person', and so on. While these statements *may* be true, donor-conceived people tell us that unless you know them to be absolutely correct, you should just stick to the facts. Why? Because many children place their biological parent on a pedestal and wait through hope-filled years for their eighteenth birthday so they can finally make a connection with this 'kind and generous' person, only to have their entire world come crashing down in a single moment when that person rejects them. So just tell your child what you know: the donor is tall with brown hair and green eyes; likes AFL football, reading romance novels and ballroom dancing . . . or whatever. As long as it's factual (hopefully).

And if you're trying to work out what kind of relationship you're going to have with the donor and siblings and you think it might look like an uncle/aunty (or other non-binary term such as auncle) and cousin kind of connection, that's great. But make sure your child understands the biological parent's true status—particularly if you're thinking you'll be able to correct any misapprehensions later when your child starts to understand, because this may have the opposite effect and suggest lies and betrayal instead.

Donor terminology

> *You don't get to dictate who a child sees as their parents. My donor is my father. I have three parents. It's up to an individual who they see as a parent.*
>
> **Australian donor-conceived adult (WA)**

For donor-conceived people, terms used for donors include, but are not limited to: their first name; 'donor'; 'sperm donor', 'egg donor' or 'embryo donor'; 'donor Dad'/'donor Mum' or other non-binary term; 'bio father/mother/parent', 'biological father/mother/parent' or 'genetic father/mother/parent'; and 'my other mother/father/parent'.

While some donor-conceived people prefer to use the term 'donor' there are many who don't because they feel it is impersonal, dehumanising or diminishes the role of their biological parent. Some people use multiple terms interchangeably depending on who they're speaking with or how they feel in the moment. Sometimes donor-conceived children raised by LGBTQIA+ parents find alternative ways to explain the donor to avoid uncomfortable and potentially upsetting questions such as 'Why don't you have a dad?' or 'Who are your "real" parents?'[226] Another consideration is that many donor-conceived people find the term 'donor' irritating because nobody donated anything to them.

> *The friction which this term* [parent] *seems to generate stems from the desire of raising parents to monopolise the term 'parent', since they are doing the parenting. This is understandable. But it is also understandable that many donor-conceived people get frustrated that they are expected to forgo acknowledging that the donor is also their biological parent.*
>
> **New Zealand sperm donor**

> *As a queer recipient parent I just want to point out that the need for a biological parent to create a child who has no romantic connection or any connection beyond the sale/ purchase of gametes, in no way alters the fact that a baby*

> *has two biological parents who may be cis or non-binary. If you don't believe me, run a DNA test. DNA doesn't lie.*
>
> **American recipient parent**

On the other hand, for recipient parents, the use of the term 'parent' is often cause for great concern and depends on how much emotional loading is brought to the word. It may be more helpful to define the word 'parent' as a noun rather than as a verb when speaking of the donor. In other words, unless you are legally co-parenting with your donor, they will not be 'parenting' your child.

Some people feel strongly that, because nouns and naming words are socially and/or legally constructed, 'parent' is not an accurate description of a donor. Some parents use several terms interchangeably when conversing with their child and allow them to arrive at a term, or terms, that work for them, and these may change over time.

Some parents use one term for describing the donor's identity to others, while their child calls the donor something else. Whatever you decide, ensure you use terminology that works for your family dynamic and, more importantly, that your child feels free to choose naming words that work for them.

> *Queer recipient parent with queer donor-conceived children here. While adults are busy getting caught up on who has a right to claim a child and the roles of raising children, most young kids are focused on biology. Donor has no real meaning to many young children. Many, in fact, teased my child for being a 'donut kid' from a 'donut dad'. Once my child ditched 'donor' for 'dad', the questions stopped altogether. It was brilliant. I wish I had known this from the start. If they try to explain donor conception, it's a lot for other kids to take in.*
>
> **American recipient parent**

Many young children struggle to describe the donor when asked by their peers so, to avoid your child doing the emotional labour, especially when they have limited vocabulary, it may be useful to work together to provide them with pre-prepared responses that work for your particular family dynamic.

Sibling terminology

> *Seeing people make up new terms for us when appropriate terms already exist feels like just another erasure and attempt to suggest that our biological relationships are different and even lesser.*
>
> **American donor-conceived adult**

Common terms to describe your donor-conceived child's siblings include 'siblings', 'sibs', 'donor sibs', 'half-siblings', 'half-brothers and sisters', 'donor brothers and sisters', or other non-binary terms where applicable.

Some donor-conceived people dislike the term 'half-sibling' because they feel that 'a sibling is a sibling' so why point out that they're only half of something. After all, people don't usually refer to their 'adopted' brother or their 'step-sister' when discussing what their family did on the weekend. Alternatively, others prefer 'half-sibling' because it helps them differentiate between the siblings they are growing up with and their donor-conceived siblings. Half-siblings can also be a useful term when the conversation is primarily about clarification and helping someone understand the relationship.

Some people use multiple terms interchangeably depending on who they're speaking with or how they feel in that moment. Of course, some donor-conceived people don't wish to acknowledge their genetic siblings at all, or feel the term is a social construct and may choose an alternative term that suits them. Again, the most important thing is to provide a variety of terms without becoming attached to any of them, or preventing the use of others. Ensure your child understands the genetic relationships, then allow them to decide what terms work best for them.

Upsetting phrases and comments

> *Being told that my donor is 'just a donor' makes my blood boil. It's so dismissive. He's not just a donor, he makes up 50%*

> *of me. I have met my donor and so much of who I am comes from him, appearance, values, attitude, temperament.*
> **Australian donor-conceived adult (ACT)**

If you've spoken to enough donor-conceived people, you will know there are certain words and phrases that can be highly irritating and, for some, can trigger extreme emotional and/or physical responses linked to a memory or situation that involved trauma.

Without the lived experience of being donor-conceived, you may see this as just a bit of silliness, but it's worth remembering that your own child may experience a similar response. Of course, they also may not. It is up to you to consider the situational context and identify whether harm is being caused through the use of any phrases or terms.

'The donor gave me a gift'

The term 'gift' has many connotations: the *gift* of life; the *gift* of gametes so recipients could become parents'; or a *gift* from God. Even so, many donor-conceived people take offence at this term. Why? Because it perpetuates the grief that some donor-conceived people experience about being given away by their biological parent and it reinforces the notion that donor-conceived children are a commodity—especially where money changed hands. Be aware that the word 'gift' can feel dehumanising. If you choose to use it, you *might* receive a response along the lines of: 'I am a human being—not a *gift* to be given.'

> *We aren't 'gifts' and we don't have to be grateful for being alive over any and all complex feelings about our existence. If you aren't 'grateful' your parents got it on in the back of a Ford Fiesta, don't come for me about my feelings on my conception.*
> **American donor-conceived adult**

'You were so loved and wanted'

Of course, there is nothing wrong with your child knowing intuitively that they were wanted but, for many donor-conceived people, hearing this verbalised can be problematic. Why? Because this statement has the potential to place an obligation of gratitude onto the child. For instance, if a child experiences emotions and feelings about their conception story that do not align with your own, they may not feel safe to speak up about their 'negative' feelings or express their genetic curiosity—they may feel invalidated. Furthermore, telling a child they were wanted relates to the fulfilment of a parent's needs and doesn't necessarily make a child feel better or special—and, in cases where the donor has rejected them, cannot be considered completely true. If you use this terminology, you may be inadvertently silencing your child and remain unaware of their true sentiments.

> *This 'wanted and loved' narrative is really problematic in donor conception—every year it is the #1 entry on lists of stuff we wish parents would stop saying to us. Better to just say 'I love you'.*
>
> **American donor-conceived adult and recipient parent**

'You should be happy to be alive'

This statement is similar to the previous statement and, again, places an obligation on the donor-conceived person to feel grateful for their existence, while simultaneously dismissing any aspects of their conception story with which they feel uncomfortable.

> *Of course I am fucking happy to be alive. No, I don't wish I had never been born. How does that, in reality, have anything to do with my thoughts and feelings around not being able to know who I am genetically? You wouldn't tell someone that's been in an accident and has injuries that they should just be happy to be alive would you? No, you would aim to provide them with support and the resources to overcome the barriers they are experiencing.*
>
> **Australian donor-conceived adult (Qld)**

'You are an angry, bitter and toxic person'

Donor-conceived people who criticise aspects of donor conception are frequently labelled as angry, bitter and toxic. Casting aspersions on vocal people is a common theme when considering marginalised groups. Like everything, a spectrum of lived experience exists and donor-conceived people sometimes even argue among themselves on social media forums where alternative views are expressed.

Nevertheless, it's important to avoid dismissing those who are courageous enough to speak up about an unethical industry, or parental behaviours that have caused them harm and to recognise that, while you may see an angry and bitter person, the reality is that this is only one aspect of their busy lives. Many donor-conceived people invest a great deal of (free) emotional labour in sharing their experiences with recipient parents, usually with the primary intention of helping them avoid the same mistakes with their children. Hearing about negative experiences can be challenging because, if we join the dots, there is an implication that our own child could feel the same way. This is, of course, an unwelcome scenario and may never eventuate, but how can we know? In any case, if you come across a vocal donor-conceived person, I urge you to see past your own discomfort and listen for the important messages that could result in healthier outcomes for your donor-conceived child.

> *Being repeatedly dismissed and told we're just angry and bitter takes its toll. Only the strongest and most passionate donor-conceived people tend to participate* [in mixed social media groups]. *And you don't NEED to hear from donor-conceived people who 'don't care'. If your child is one of those people, then you won't have to do anything and there's nothing to prepare for. But why wouldn't you want to be prepared for the alternative?*
>
> **Australian donor-conceived adult (NSW)**

'The donor-conceived people on those social media groups are not representative of all donor-conceived people'

This comment is bandied about with regularity and in a similar fashion to the previous comment, is designed to highlight that many donor-conceived people do not experience any problems with their conception story. While this is true (and we all, no doubt, hope this scenario describes our own children) it is important to acknowledge that, even when only small numbers of people express grief and trauma, change is needed.

> *It's a shame how much donor-conceived people's feelings are painted as black and white (you're okay with your conception or you're not, you're positive/well-adjusted or you're not). There is so much to donor conception, people have complex thoughts about a complex topic and those thoughts change over time. Nothing is simple about this, and that's okay.*
>
> **American donor-conceived adult**

'Perhaps you just need therapy'

This statement is regularly thrown about in forums where donor-conceived people speak up about their experiences. While the reality is that many donor-conceived people do undergo or have undergone therapy, this kind of uninvited solution to all one's problems is dismissive and invalidates a person's lived experience. Speaking up about feelings and emotions is healthy and, if commentary from a donor-conceived person makes you feel uncomfortable, there *might* be something of value for you to explore in that. It's also important to be aware that a donor-conceived person who tells you they're 'happy' could be withholding their true feelings in order to protect their parents or others.

> *You can be a happy, well-adjusted human with a successful, productive life and still take issue with the way you were conceived and the industry that helped your creation.*
>
> **Australian donor-conceived adult (WA)**

15
Donor and Sibling Linking

Love is not zero sum. There's not less for you because someone else gets some. If you think it's possible to love more than two children, consider that it is also possible to love more than two parents.

American donor-conceived adult

Donor and sibling linking refers to the process by which people in the donor conception triad (donor-conceived people, donors and recipient parents) identify and connect with each other. In the early days of donor conception, recipient parents were unlikely to discover who their donor was and the donor-conceived children would have no knowledge of, or subsequent access to, donor siblings. With the availability of donor IDs, direct-to-consumer DNA testing and social media, things are very different today. But does a genetic connection even equate to 'family'? How does one navigate this strange, unknown territory and the concept of multiple strangers (in some cases, hundreds) connecting simply because people chose the same donor?

Considerable variation has been observed between donor-conceived people regarding the importance they place on their biological parent and siblings. Some donor-conceived people attribute little significance to connecting with a biological parent, but place great importance on finding siblings. Some join sibling groups but don't participate; others develop lasting relationships with their siblings. Some people consider both the donor and siblings as important, while others care for neither and don't believe that genetics equates to kinship. Some individuals fully embrace the connections they've made with the donor and the donor's extended family, while others have shared that they don't wish to be as close to the donor as others expect them to be.[227] Some donor-conceived people simply wish to understand genetic resemblances or identify important medical information without having a relationship with the donor. Others describe the process of 'hunting their biological parent down', silently observing them on social media before deciding whether or not to make contact, while simultaneously trying to identify what it is that they do want from them—be it a one-off meeting, a relationship, medical information . . .

> *It's not homophobic nor transphobic to say that every human deserves basic rights to their identity. Queer folk are uniquely positioned to embrace a model of family creation that steps outside heteronormativity. We don't need to estrange our children from their genetic identity to embrace our identities. From a Queer, genderqueer BIPOC recipient parent.*
>
> **American recipient parent**

In a 2020 survey conducted on 481 donor-conceived people from countries around the world:[228] 88% of the respondents expressed the belief that it is a basic human right to know the identity of both one's biological parents; 90% considered it important to know their genetic siblings; and 71% of participants agreed with the statement: 'The method of my conception sometimes causes me to feel distressed, angry, or sad.'

Despite surveys such as this being small in scope and participants often being self-selected, the existence of many worldwide support groups for donor-conceived teens and adults, websites, social media groups, workshops for donor-conceived children, research studies, and more, offer further evidence that many donor-conceived people do wish to connect with their biological relatives.

> *Donor-conceived people being interested in our genetics is seen as a heteronormative 'preoccupation' when in fact for many of us, it's essential to feel whole, and if it looks like an obsession, maybe that is just because it has been denied to us. It's probably very hard for most people to understand because they take knowing their genetic relatives for granted.*
>
> **American donor-conceived adult**

And is it even necessary to understand why people are interested in their biological ties? As donor-conceived adult Rzeka stated:

> *It's not just academics. There are a variety of actors who assert that the desire to know one's biological parent(s) is pathological or a result of heteronormative socialization that must be 'unlearned' . . . Trying to find the reason why donor-conceived adults want to know their genetic families is futile and unethical and it's about time somebody said it.*[229]

Emotions and feelings, like most things in life, evolve over time and your child's interest in their biological parent and siblings is likely to ebb and flow. But even so, the three messages consistently heard from large numbers of donor-conceived people are: the desire to be informed about their origins; the need for information about their biological parent and siblings; and the possibility of connecting with their genetic relatives, should they wish to do so.

Regardless, without access to the information that outlines their genetic origins, donor-conceived people are deprived of the ability to determine the level of importance of this for themselves. 'Genealogical bewilderment' is a condition that can follow, a term that refers to identity issues and the corresponding anxiety experienced by people who have little or no knowledge of their biological parent(s).

Child or parent-led?

> *Child led practices are misunderstood. It doesn't mean waiting till they choose something they have no experience with. It means creating the experiences and relationships, so they can choose to opt in or out once they know what they can choose. It's up to the adults to facilitate it. Imagine never introducing your child to a grandparent and then wondering why your thirteen year old has no interest in grandma at the family reunion.*
>
> **Australian recipient parent**

> *That's a responsibility* [asking to meet siblings and bio-parents] *that doesn't belong on a child's shoulders. Should we wait until the child can speak in full sentences before we introduce them to family and friends?*
>
> **American donor-conceived person**

Many people experience complicated or unpleasant relationships with their biological family. Some people choose estrangement; others have it imposed upon them by family members who reject aspects of their lifestyle—for example, sexuality or expressions of gender identity. The LGBTQIA+ community has spent many years fighting for the right just to have a legally recognised family, including access to donor gametes, child adoption, and legal recognition as non-biological parents.

In any scenario, the rejection or loss of family can be painful and devastating. As a result, many people find themselves in the position of choosing their own family; people who are not genetically related but meet personal definitions of 'family' that include important elements such as love, respect and support—chosen family is crucial for many LGBTQIA+ people.

Your own experience with biological family notwithstanding, it's important to avoid the presumption that your donor-conceived child will prioritise their biological relationships in the same way as you. Donor-conceived children need to be given the space to explore their feelings and make their own decisions about their genetic connections. In other words, your child can't make a decision to step away from something (or someone) they don't know exists. So, if you are thinking of leaving the decision to your child to meet their siblings when they're ready, not only are you placing a huge amount of emotional labour on them to speak up and make the connections happen, you are also actually making a decision for them. As one ten-year-old Australian donor-conceived child put it:

> *I'm so glad I've never had to 'meet' the donor. I've known him my whole life. I'd be scared about meeting him now.*

Love and genetics are both important—one doesn't need to negate the other.

Connecting with the donor

> *I've got close to ten little humans in my life as a result of donating my eggs. I'm Auntie A to all of them. I have a loving relationship with all but one (one family has made a parental choice not to prioritise their child's needs). It's the absolute best—and should be the norm—when you have time to explore and develop emotional connections and a relationship with children you're related to. Many donor-conceived adults have indicated to me that they would have preferred access to all of their biological family during their formative years. It's important to consider the needs of donor-conceived individuals and prioritise those needs over the comfort of their parents.*
>
> **Australian known egg donor**

Reaching out to your donor

> *Initially, before I found my bio-father Glen, I was driven mad with questions. That was the biggest thing, the not knowing and also the not knowing when, or if, I would ever know. But when I found him that then shifted to fear of being rejected. This did not eventuate, thankfully. He has been warm, welcoming and generous. But his children and his sister don't want to know about me. They don't want to meet me. Like I am some shit on their shoe—some stupid thing Glen did when he was twenty-one.*
>
> **Australian donor-conceived adult (WA)**

As a parent, the notion of reaching out and connecting with the donor who contributed to the creation of your child tends to evoke a range of emotions—fear and trepidation, excitement and hope—a veritable emotional (and ethical) minefield.

Oh, what to do! The questions are many, the answers unknown and unpredictable. Should I, in the case of anonymous or ID release donors, try to find them? Is making contact with the donor the right thing to do? Will I upset the donor and their family? Did the donor even tell their family (and kids) about their donations? Will the donor reject my child or, alternatively, will they seek a co-parenting arrangement and shared parental responsibility? Will the donor accept my child if they find out they've been raised by LGBTQIA+ parents?[230] Will I get sued by the sperm or egg bank? Do I need my child's consent before reaching out? Will the other families who used the same donor reject us if I reach out—should I ask all of them for consent first? Will the donor even be alive if my child has to wait eighteen years? Should I listen to the voices of family, friends and social media 'experts' who tell me I have no right to 'invade the donor's privacy'? Which will I regret more: reaching out and being rejected; or waiting and receiving a 'We wish you'd made contact a long time ago!' response?

Whatever choices you make, attempting to connect with donors and siblings will involve some effort and, depending on your situation, will require making contact with your clinic, completing an application to your state or territory's donor register (see 'Donor registers and recordkeeping' later in this chapter), contacting your sperm or egg bank, doing some social media sleuthing, or using a direct-to-consumer DNA test to test your child.

Of course, every situation is different and many questions cannot be answered until you take action. In any case, reaching out requires an act of bravery. Perhaps the most important part of your decision-making process involves defining whose needs are the most important in the great debate; those of your clinic, your bank, your donor, the donor's family, the other families who used your donor—or your child?

Writing a letter/message

The words you use to reach out to your donor and the method by which you do so will be unique to you and your situation. Consider what you need to say and, if your child is old enough, what *they* might like to say.

Following are some tips to help you.

Note: The suggestions below have been gathered from counsellors, donors and donor-conceived people.

- Consider speaking with a qualified counsellor before going ahead with contact attempts.
- Keep it simple to start with and see what the donor's reaction is (avoid a long essay).
- Unless you know otherwise, assume the donor knows nothing about their donor-conceived children, especially if there are a large number of siblings. Do not refer to any children *other than your own* in your initial message.
- Thank the donor for the part they've played in building your family.
- Avoid being overly 'gushy' with your wording.
- Write a few drafts and take your time over the message until you feel comfortable to send it.
- Keep photos to a minimum or, if you don't feel comfortable sending photos, you might wish to ask the donor if they would like to see some.
- Outline what it is you are seeking in both the short-term and the long-term. For example, a short-term goal might be to establish some intermittent contact, including being able to ask questions as your child raises them. A long-term goal might be meeting face-to-face at a mutually agreed time in the future.
- Be patient. Sometimes donors need time to process the fact that they have created children. They may also need to share with their family the news about you having made contact. Some families report waiting months before they receive a response from their donor.
- While considering the possibility that the donor will welcome contact, be prepared for the possibility that they will not. Have support processes in place for your child either way.

Note: If your older child wishes to contact their biological parent by themselves, it may be beneficial for them to seek counselling with an appropriately qualified person before going ahead. They can also join the Donor Conceived Australia and We Are Donor Conceived groups for support from other donor-conceived people. (See 'Useful tools and resources' at the back of this book for links to online sources containing additional resources, blog articles and the latest updates, including information about these groups.)

Connecting with siblings and their families

> *Don't wait for the kids to ask. They may never ask. When I was a child, I pretended to not care at all about my biological family. I felt the need to protect my parents' feelings. I don't believe that it should be child-led. My parents never asked if I wanted to meet my cousins, grandparents, aunts and uncles. They never waited for me to express interest and say that I wanted to know them. Family is family, and there's no need to wait, even if it is a different version of family than any of you are used to.*
>
> **American donor-conceived adult**

> *Known donor to a queer couple here—baby has met me, my family, we have catch ups every few months. The amount of medical and personality info they've gotten from me and my family is huge already. Big things like allergies to anaesthesia and little things like tips for eczema. He's like a nephew to me, I have zero interest in being a mother or 'taking' him, we follow the lead of his parents in terms of contact. It's lovely and puts the baby first. We're ready for the child to choose more or less contact as he grows up so he has some control over his life.*
>
> **Australian egg donor**

For donor-conceived people, the importance of connections with siblings varies enormously, just as it does for their connections with a biological parent. Some have no desire to know or meet their siblings, while others express interest from a very young age. An Australian donor-conceived adult explains:

> *There are all kinds of issues at play. But it is valid to deal with the difficulties of being donor-conceived by just shutting them out, if that's what you choose to! It's definitely painful for other siblings, etc. to be rejected but, of course, we all have the right to choose not to pursue relationships for any reason.*

Another Australian donor-conceived person describes their experience:

> *I don't think there are any guaranteed solutions. Much depends on the individual's personality and approach to life. I have siblings who care greatly about being donor-conceived and some who don't seem to think too much about it. I have one full brother who prefers to ignore it totally—to the point where he has continued to play out a charade of creating a false narrative for himself that includes updating our inaccurate family tree for his children and refusing to meet our new sibs.*

An Australian donor-conceived adult from NSW says:

> *There is a definite stage where it is all too much and you feel numb about everything. It comes and goes and then comes back again when you feel as if you can't give everyone what they want—or if they don't seem to care as much as you do. This is why it is so much work to build these relationships as adults and why we should grow up knowing everyone.*

Some donor-conceived people feel it's a safer option reaching out to siblings rather than their biological parent because the siblings are in the same situation as them. Many donor-conceived adults express disappointment and anger about not being given the opportunity to connect with their siblings as children, lamenting the years that can never be retrieved and describing awkward meetings as adults. Some share great delight in connecting with the donor's own children, while others find themselves being rejected by those siblings.

Donor-conceived siblings are the best part of donor conception. If you insist on having a donor-conceived kid, at the very least connect them to their family.

Donor-conceived teenager (13 years old)

A 2020 study of forty-seven donor-conceived people in their twenties, all of whom were conceived using ID Release donors, showed that almost all participants expressed curiosity and interest towards their donor-conceived siblings. Motivations seemed to stem from a desire to understand who they themselves were as individuals, personal identity creation and finding 'people like me', as well as forming relationships with those genetically-related people. Some individuals described connecting with siblings as having 'less risk' than connecting with their biological parent.[231]

Sometimes having connections with other donor-conceived children, even when they're not related, can help to normalise children's conception stories. In LGBTQIA+ communities this tends to occur naturally. Many SMC/SPC families also create communities and connect with other donor-conceived families. Heterosexual families, on the other hand, tend to do so less regularly.

How to make contact

If you are in any local donor-conceived groups or even parenting groups you can just ask 'anyone with donor-conceived kids fancy meeting up?' My kid enjoyed going to those types of events at a park or the beach when younger. Mostly the kids did not actually talk about being donor-conceived. For mine it was enough to know the other kids were donor-conceived, to not be alone in the world as something strange. Meeting siblings is special.

Australian recipient parent

So what are the processes related to recordkeeping and donor conception? Who is the holder of this sacred information and how do people access it? How do you make contact with your donor-conceived child's siblings, their parents, or your donor?

The answers vary depending on the type of donor you select and, if you choose an Australian clinic-recruited donor, it also depends on the state or territory and the clinic in which you undergo treatment.

Donor registers and recordkeeping

Recordkeeping

Since the introduction of the Reproductive Technology Accreditation Committee (RTAC), one of the RTAC's most fundamental principles is that recipient parents and their children are to be given the most important consideration in all decisions and that children have the right to know their genetic origins.[232] Accordingly, the National Health and Medical Research Council's *Ethical Guidelines* outline the responsibilities that clinics have regarding recordkeeping. These responsibilities involve (but are not limited to) ensuring that data reporting complies with any relevant Commonwealth, state or territory legislation, and that the names and contact details of all parties involved in ART procedures at the clinic are recorded along with, where possible, the names of any children born. It also involves making sure that this information is available to those same parties.[233]

What is a donor register?

A donor register is where information is held about the donor and the birth details of the donor-conceived child, as well as the person undergoing ART treatment. Clinics provide the relevant information to the register (if one exists) after the children are born. The state or territory in which you *undergo* ART treatment (not the state in which you *reside*) will determine which register holds the records.

Other naming conventions may be used to refer to the donor register, such as 'central register', 'database', or others. Check to see whether a register is in place in your local jurisdiction.

Once a donor-conceived person reaches the requisite age (this might vary depending on the state or territory), identifying information about the donor may be made available to them. Rules regarding the access to information by others, (such as parents, donors and siblings) may also apply. Check to determine what rules apply in your jurisdiction.

If you undergo ART treatment in a state or territory where there is no donor register, your clinic must ensure all relevant information is recorded and will be available for release to donors, recipient parents and to the donor-conceived people born.[234]

Voluntary registers

A voluntary register is an information sharing and linking service, through which it may be possible for you or your child to access information about the donor and/or siblings at a much younger age. Check to see whether a voluntary register exists in your local jurisdiction.

Other naming conventions may be used and the voluntary register might operate separately from the standard donor register in your jurisdiction, or the two registers could be combined.

A voluntary register enables donors, parents, donor-conceived people (and possibly relatives of donor-conceived people) to provide information about themselves at any age with the intention of either obtaining information or making contact with other genetic family members. For example, an application for contact with other siblings or the donor might be made by a parent as soon as their child is born. Not all families may wish to connect and, consequently, both parties must express interest and consent to sharing information before a connection might be arranged.

Where no such register exists, clinics can take on the exchange of information between relevant parties, although clinics may have slightly different systems in place. For instance, some clinics have an online linking system for families and donors, while other clinics allow recipient parents to write letters to their donor which they then pass on. So, while clinics must help parents understand the significance of biological connections and provide them with a supportive environment within which to meet the donor and siblings,[235] depending on the local jurisdiction they may not be compelled to actually connect anyone. This could impact your child's ability to connect with their siblings and the donor from a young age, so make sure you check this with the clinic before you start treatment. Your child may thank you for it one day.

> ***Note:*** Donor registers are constantly evolving and may have different functions or operate differently in each state and territory. Check what applies in your local jurisdiction. It's also important to know that donor registers are dependent upon the quality and availability of records.[236]

Recordkeeping with an international donor

If you choose an international donor via an Australian clinic, all records of the treatment procedures and the people involved (yourself, your donor and your donor-conceived child) will be held at the Australian clinic. Your donor's identifying information arrives in Australia along with their gametes. If you undergo treatment in a state or territory that has a donor register, the clinic is also required to pass this information on to the donor register.

The international agency or bank *should* also keep a record of all relevant parties but the processes involved will vary depending on the country and the bank you select. They should also keep a record of all of your child's siblings but, unfortunately, it's possible that your child may never be able to locate or communicate with your ID Release donor, or some of their half-siblings, or even identify how many siblings they have.

Furthermore, the extent to which a bank or agency maintains contact with your donor, and the related policies around this, may vary considerably. It is not uncommon for international banks or agencies to never communicate with their donors again once they have completed their donations.

If you undergo ART treatment in another country, recordkeeping and subsequent release of information will be dictated by the legislation (if any) and policies of your chosen country. Given that many countries offer anonymous donors only, this means your child may never gain access to the identifying details of their biological parent unless they undergo a direct-to-consumer DNA test.

Recordkeeping with a known donor

Known donor and a fertility clinic

If you choose a known donor and undergo ART treatment at an Australian clinic, all records of the treatment procedures and the people involved (yourself, your known donor and your donor-conceived child) are the responsibility of the clinic. If you undergo treatment in a state or territory that has a donor register, the clinic is required to pass this information on to that register as per the relevant protocol.

Known donors and 'at-home' insemination

If you choose a known donor and complete AI at home (or at another location), it may be possible to record your details on the donor register voluntarily. Check the rules that apply in your local jurisdiction.

In terms of contact between yourself, your donor and your donor-conceived child, you get to make the rules. (For more information about co-parenting and parental rights and responsibilities see Chapter 6, 'Known Donors', and Chapter 16, 'ART Regulations and Ethical Guidelines').

Bank or agency linking sites

If you use an international donor, irrespective of the Australian state or territory in which you undergo ART treatment, you can attempt to make contact with other parents around the globe who have used the same donor. In fact, you may be able to make contact *prior to* selecting your international donor, so you can check with other parents about their experience of using that donor (see Chapter 10, 'Further Research Tips for Selecting Clinics, Countries and Donors').

Some sperm and egg banks also have their own voluntary registers which enable people to find other parents who have used the same donor and who wish to connect. In some cases, the donor may also choose to join the register. Donor-conceived children *may* also be able to join when they are old enough.

Banks will not usually allow people to join their linking sites until they have registered the child's birth. They tend to monitor their sites very carefully and are likely to have visibility of all messages between users. Many people use these sites to find other families and then, to ensure more privacy, quickly create their own private groups on social media platforms.

If you are using an international donor, check whether the sperm or egg bank has a linking site. In rare cases, the bank may also pass on a message to your donor indicating that you wish to connect. Currently, however, many banks refuse to do this.

Independent linking sites

An independent linking site is a platform that is not associated with any sperm or egg banks, egg agencies or clinics—the Donor Sibling Registry[237] is currently the largest site available. The main purpose of independent linking sites is to assist people to find their families but, in some instances they can also be useful for uncovering information prior to conception. For instance, you may be able to enquire how many existing children your potential donor has, or whether the sperm or egg bank you are about to use has a reputation for large numbers of donor siblings, and so on.

Independent linking sites operate slightly differently from each other but, generally, they require you to provide information such as your Donor's ID, and the bank and clinic used. In some cases you can also include a paragraph about yourself, your child, what kind of connection you are seeking, and any other details you believe to be relevant. Anyone on the site who has used the same donor and wishes to respond to you will do so. Most people then choose another social media platform, such as a private Facebook group, to continue the relationship.

Many thousands of families have successfully connected via linking sites (my family included), although it's important to know that sometimes Donor IDs are incorrect and people who believe they are siblings discover after completing a DNA test that they are not.

Sometimes people enter their information on linking sites and then choose not to communicate. This can be confusing and upsetting for other people seeking to make connections, so make sure you are clear about your intentions before entering your information on a linking site.

Some sites cost money to join and have ongoing fees each year. Others are free. Some sites require you to provide a significant amount of your personal information. Do your homework and make sure you're completely comfortable with the site before handing over your money and your private details. (See 'Useful tools and resources' at the back of this book for links to online sources containing additional resources, blog articles and the latest updates, including more information about independent linking sites.)

Social media

> *I believe I have an obligation to my donor-conceived children to make myself available, especially about medical issues. On the other hand, if they don't want to know me, I have to accept that.*
>
> **Australian sperm donor**

Social media groups can help you decide which is the right clinic, bank, country or donor, but they can also be useful for linking you to your child's siblings and, in some cases, to your donor. For instance, there are many Facebook groups discussing the topic of donor conception and some of these groups have a pinned post at the top where a donor's ID can be added. Alternatively, the online group might prefer you to send your donor's ID to the administrator for a more discreet way of determining matches—this is also because matches, on occasions, may turn out to be incorrect where donor IDs have been duplicated or 'fiddled' with.

Some families set up private searchable Facebook groups with names that incorporate the donor's ID—although many of these require you to have had a donor-conceived child before you can join. So, a general search of Facebook may help you discover information about your potential donor.

A Google search using your donor's ID and photos may also provide results, as well as other reverse image and facial recognition search engines (particularly if the donor has used the same photo for their donor profile and their social media page). Some of these search engines may require a fee.

These days many donors are keen to make a connection with their donor-conceived children/adults and some have even been known to create YouTube channels using their Donor ID as part of the channel name.

Some banks and fertility clinics have their own social media pages, enabling you to check whether anyone else has used your donor and to connect directly in this way. Alternatively, recipient parents may have set up a group run independently by the parents, but which incorporates the name of the clinic.

If you are considering a known donor via a matching site and the matching site has a forum for conversations, you can ask whether there's an existing private group set up for the families who have conceived using that donor.

In all cases, before making a post on any online platform, ensure you read the rules of the social media group—including lists of terms considered offensive. Take some time to read through existing posts to develop a sense of the group's general tone and atmosphere—and don't post your donor's ID on the site unless you are permitted to do so.

Direct-to-consumer DNA testing

> *All sorts of information comes to light when people DNA test. I see many Not Parent Expected (NPE) events—donor conception, rape, incest, double cousins. When people ask me to search for them, I have to make sure they're prepared to deal with the results.*
>
> **Emma-Lee Still (Australian genetic genealogist and egg donor)**

Completing DNA tests is another means by which siblings and donors can locate and connect with each other and for some, particularly those who use anonymous donors, it may be the only way.

More and more people are discovering via direct-to-consumer DNA testing that they are donor-conceived. So, don't be the parent who holds their breath during the television commercials when vibrant actors announce, 'There could be more to your story! Pay today and receive a 20% discount on your DNA test!'

Because so many people are DNA testing these days, a person can often be found and identified even if they have not completed a test themselves. If half-siblings have tested, this can assist with narrowing down results. As more people offer up their DNA for testing, locating relatives will become easier.

What is direct-to-consumer DNA testing?

Most genetic testing for such things as inheritable disorders or for predicting the risks of specific conditions is carried out by a professional in a healthcare centre, but the introduction of direct-to-consumer genetic DNA testing has opened up new possibilities for finding relatives. It's also cheap and easy, but what is it exactly?

Genetic or DNA test kits are usually purchased online and involve sending a cheek swab or a saliva sample to a laboratory (depending on the DNA company's requirements). Extraneous material, such as cell debris and proteins, is removed and the DNA is extracted and analysed by a computer program that estimates ancestral makeup by assigning specific percentages (for example, 22% European). Is the process perfect and fully understood? No. Are there system limitations? Yes.

And as more people undergo testing and more data is gathered, personal results may change over time.[238] In some countries DNA testing is not allowed so, despite many recipient parents believing otherwise, there is no guarantee an anonymous donor will be found.

Is it safe to undergo a direct-to-consumer DNA test?

> *The DNA companies know that trust is paramount because otherwise share prices will plummet. Security and trust is their business.*
>
> **Emma-Lee Still (Australian genetic genealogist and egg donor)**

As is true of the fertility industry, DNA testing is also big business and the jury is out as to whether sending your DNA off to a commercial enterprise is placing you, or your child, at risk—or what the exact nature of that risk might be. The NHMRC recommends that Australians exercise caution when DNA testing and consider the implications, not just for themselves but for other family members as well.[239]

One of the first things to do if you're planning to DNA test your child is to read the fine print to determine exactly what you are signing up for and what scenarios you are able to opt in or out of. For example, will your child's data be on-sold to a pharmaceutical company and then possibly on-sold again? If you discover a health condition, will this impact your life insurance or income protection insurance? Other steps you can take are to avoid small DNA testing companies you've never heard of, review the company's privacy policy and ensure the company is accredited to worldwide standards.

Should you DNA test your child?

> *There's no way I'd DNA test my child. I believe genetic testing should only be done by a consenting adult, a person who can truly understand the potential outcomes of handing over their DNA to a global for-profit organisation.*
>
> **Australian recipient parent**

> *In general, I think the DNA companies are more ethically responsible than commercial sperm banks. If you purchased genetic material from a company that is primarily concerned about profit, you can upload your child's DNA to a database to help find the source of their genetics. It's a bit sci-fi but that's just donor-conceived life.*
>
> **Erin Jackson (founder of We Are Donor Conceived)**

Whether you DNA test your child or not is a very personal decision and, for many, poses quite the ethical dilemma. Some people test their child shortly after birth; others feel the need to wait until their child is old enough to provide informed consent. When DNA testing minors, there are certain safety precautions you can put in place, such as: using non-identifying email addresses and user names; and keeping family trees private. When you first make contact with matches, it may be worthwhile skirting carefully around the issue of donor conception and taking screenshots of new high matches and their shared matches in case those matches subsequently hide their profile from you. In other words, don't assume that because someone is on a DNA site that they are ready to be found. The other factor to consider is whether you're really ready to connect with your child's genetically-related families—if another family reaches out, are you going to reject contact? If so, that could be very confusing for the other party, so make sure you're clear about your intentions moving forward.

How do I do it?

> *DNA results are heavily skewed towards European history because the majority of people testing are of European origin.*
>
> **Emma-Lee Still (Australian genetic genealogist and egg donor)**

The bigger the DNA company is, the more matches you are likely to have on the site. If the site requires a saliva test, it may be challenging to test small babies, but it is not beyond the realms of possibility. Other sites require swab tests, and these tests are far easier for young children to undergo. Some sites also allow you to upload the raw DNA data from other testing companies, which means you get better value and you could match with more people.

If you need assistance finding someone, there are many wonderful 'DNA Detectives' and 'Search Angels' willing to help you for free on various social media sites.

Will I be sued by my sperm bank?

While many people fear they will be sued by their sperm bank, it's important to know that, at the time of writing this book, no sperm bank has ever sued a recipient parent for testing their child's DNA. Much of this fear of litigation seems to originate with the 2019 USA case,

Teuscher v CCB-NWB, LLC.[240] But this case is frequently misquoted and it was the recipient parent who sued, not the sperm bank. In this case, the recipient parent (Danielle Teuscher), made contact with the donor's mother, someone complained to the sperm bank and the bank subsequently denied Teuscher access to her remaining sperm vials. Teuscher sued the sperm bank and received US$75,000 in an out-of-court settlement.[241]

So, if you have not yet completed your family, a DNA test may be worth putting on hold in case your sperm bank behaves in a similar manner to the one in the case described. Check the sperm/egg bank's donor contract, if one exists.

Risks of donor and sibling linking

> *My son has lots of siblings, both here and overseas, and one of the families is pretty unpleasant (I won't go into details). I have zero interest in meeting them and the thought of my son being influenced by them is a bit scary. Anyway, the fact remains that my kid and their kid are brothers, so when they're old enough they can work out if they want to know each other. In the meantime, I'll just remain polite and keep the conversation open. Which is easy thankfully, because they live in another state.*
>
> **Australian recipient parent**

Despite the wonderful connections that can be made with biological parents and siblings, it doesn't always work out—sometimes there can be sadness or trauma when reality doesn't meet expectations. For instance, sometimes donor-conceived people are rejected by their biological parents (and vice versa), or siblings are not interested in meeting. Occasionally recipient parents just can't relate to each other, or vast political, religious or cultural gaps exist that cannot be bridged. Sometimes it may even feel unsafe to connect with another family.

In any case, it's important to consider the needs of your child, and the fact that this is *their* story and that, later, their choices could be different from yours. When they reach their teens or adulthood, they may wish to contact or re-establish connections with siblings or the donor (even if you don't like the families). So, try to leave pathways open for your child to do whatever they wish to do in the future.

For scenarios in which your child has experienced rejection from a biological parent, grandparent, sibling or other, or where interactions elicit complex emotions, it may be prudent to seek assistance for your child in the form of a counsellor experienced in the nuances of donor conception.

Bear in mind that there is also the possibility you were provided with different gametes than the ones you chose and a false match might result. Direct-to-consumer DNA testing is the only way to guarantee genetic connections.

Legal Implications

> *As it is for all children, it is E's* [the child's] *best interests that are by law the paramount concern of the Court. It is not what is fair to the various adults around him. And although parents and carers naturally have hopes and dreams for their children, and the right to make many fundamental choices and decisions as to how they will be raised, if their hopes or choices collide with the child's best interests, it is the latter that must prevail.*
>
> **Excerpt from the court judgement of *Wilson & Roberts* [2010]**[242]

Some recipient parents feel nervous about the possibility of connecting with their donor too early or too frequently, especially those who have used known donors or clinic-recruited donors. Why? Because Australian Family Law has lagged behind donor-linking laws and, in some situations, connecting may introduce legal implications (see Chapter 16, 'ART Regulations and Ethical Guidelines'). For instance, if a donor builds a relationship with a child, that donor could potentially gain legal rights.

A court will consider such factors as: how conception occurred; what is set out in any agreement made; whether the donor was registered on the birth certificate; whether the donor and the recipient parent had a previous relationship; any financial contributions made; regularity of contact; and how the child identifies with the donor.

If you are considering known donation, it's absolutely essential that you and your donor both feel informed and agree on all matters; this includes expressing and agreeing upon where you stand regarding both current and future scenarios.

Balancing the rights of your child with the rights of the donor is a complex and challenging undertaking. Have you discussed every conceivable situation and how you might respond in the event that any of those situations unfold? Are there any circumstances in which either of you might be able to say, 'Oh, I didn't know!' or 'I didn't think that through'?

Once you have worked through all of these points, you can then document everything in a preconception agreement. Working through this process with a family lawyer is a good idea. And while you may choose to avoid options such as using an ex-partner as your donor or avoiding financial contributions and, conversely, getting to know your donor and establishing trust, at the end of the day should a dispute arise, a court will always decide in the best interests of the child.

Part Seven:
The Law and Other Guidelines

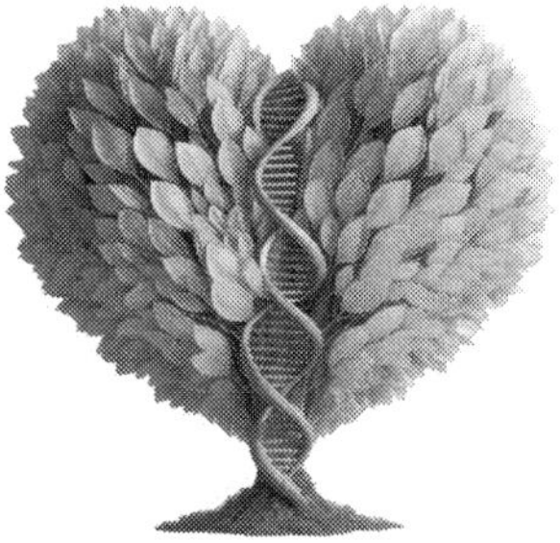

People and families are complex. No two situations are ever the same. Law attempts to deal with them all, but of course it can most definitely struggle to keep up with science and the resulting changes in societal norms and values. This particular area of law really is a prime example of that.

The best advice I can give anyone entering this world is to be open, honest, and to own your decisions. Arm yourself with knowledge early on and at all ages and stages of your child's life. Obtain appropriate legal advice, at various stages as necessary, which is tailored to individual circumstances and which can be relied upon. Record contemporaneous intentions, and formalise agreements which comply with the law of your jurisdiction and, importantly, which do not contradict it. As with any parenting journey,

> *be prepared for ANYTHING! Ensure that the best interests of your child always remain the paramount consideration in any decision making. This is the best way to protect your child and to avoid great emotional and financial cost (and, ideally, lawyers) in the future.*
>
> *As Maya Angelou said, 'Do the best you can until you know better. Then when you know better, do better.*[243]
>
> **Courtney du Toit**
> **(Australian family lawyer and donor-conceived adult)**

While the legal implications surrounding donor conception might feel a little yawn-inducing, there are some important things you need to know, especially if you're considering a known donor. Frequent questions that arise include: 'How do I register my child's birth when I've used a donor?'; 'Will I be the legal parent?'; 'Will the *donor* be a legal parent?'; 'Should I obtain a preconception agreement and, if so, does it actually mean anything?'

The following chapter will answer all of those questions and more.

Note: The information discussed in this chapter, unless otherwise stated, describes Australian legislation and ethical guidelines. If you are travelling to a foreign country to undergo ART treatment, it is highly recommended you research the relevant jurisdiction's legislation, if any exists, and consider how that may impact you and your child.

16

ART Regulations and Ethical Guidelines

It may surprise you to know that there is currently no Commonwealth legislation in Australia that specifically regulates ART. This is because regulation of health matters, including ART, falls to the individual states. The *Family Law Act 1975* (Cth) intersects with state legislation, such as the *Status of Children Act*(s) which individually deal with legal parentage in the respective Australian states. Where conflict arises, Commonwealth law generally prevails. All states have their own legislation related to birth certificates, legal parentage and embryo research.

Anonymity

> *I felt a loss that I couldn't give my child that history and knowledge, like it was some form of failing as his mum. It hurt when my child asked, and when I had to explain why he did not have a grandfather. Anonymity has an intergenerational impact on donor-conceived families, it takes away from the identity of multiple generations.*
>
> **Australian donor-conceived adult (Qld)**

Once upon a time, in a manner similar to adoptive parents, parents of donor-conceived children were counselled to keep such matters secret. Sometimes this was expressed quite literally as, 'Go home, have sex and forget this ever happened.' With the availability of direct-to-consumer DNA testing, anonymity can no longer be guaranteed. However, perhaps somewhat pointlessly, many foreign countries still offer anonymity and seek to enforce it (at least for a period of time).

We now know through research and experience that full disclosure generally provides better outcomes for donor-conceived people[244] (see Chapter 14, 'Talking about Donor Conception'). As a result, the guidelines regarding donor anonymity have changed in Australia and all donors must now consent to ID Release status.[245]

While donor anonymity has been banned by several other countries, including (but not limited to) New Zealand, the UK, Sweden, Austria, Germany, Switzerland, the Netherlands, Norway, Uruguay and Ireland, there are still many countries that continue to offer this option, in some instances promoting it as 'the best way to make a child truly yours'.

In many countries, donor anonymity is the *only* option available. Anonymity means fertility clinics and banks are subject to less scrutiny and it may even enable them to hide behind substandard practices. Interestingly, many donors express that they don't wish to be anonymous, but that it is the only option being presented to them.

Some countries are allowing people to indicate a preference for open donation when they undergo ART treatment and, if both parties agree, there is the possibility of contact—but that is never guaranteed.

If an Australian fertility specialist promotes or recommends overseas travel to access anonymous donor gametes, they are in breach of the NHMRC *Ethical Guidelines*.[246]

Fertility clinics

Australian fertility clinics offering ART treatment must comply with Commonwealth legislation, as well as any existing state legislation. Their practices are also required to comply with the RTAC *Code of Practice* and the NHMRC *Ethical Guidelines* (see Chapter 7, 'Choosing an Australian Fertility Clinic').

If a clinic is shown to be noncompliant, assessment of any incident is carried out in the following order:

1. the relevant Commonwealth legislation prevails over state legislation; then
2. the relevant state legislation prevails over the RTAC *Code of Practice* and the NHMRC *Ethical Guidelines*.[247]

In some states, government regulatory bodies (such as VARTA in Victoria[248]) also monitor clinics and have various roles related to compliance. Other government bodies that can also play a part in assisting with regulatory functions related to ART activities include (but are not limited to) the Australian Health Practitioner Regulation Agency (APHRA) and the Australian Competition and Consumer Commission (ACCC).

Where serious breaches occur (such as intentionally using excess embryos for research without authorisation;[249] undergoing training with fertilisation procedures where the individual does not have a licence to do so;[250] or giving or receiving payment for the supply of a human egg, human sperm or a human embryo[251]) the breaches will likely result in clinics being held accountable in a court of law and subject to hefty fines, or could even result in imprisonment for the offending individuals.

Can a clinic provide ART treatment without RTAC accreditation?

Clinics are legally prevented from providing ART treatment without RTAC accreditation. Australian clinics that carry out ART treatment involving donated gametes or embryos and IUI must have an RTAC licence. If a clinic is providing ART treatment without an RTAC licence, they are in breach of the law—including the *Research Involving Human Embryos Act 2002* (Cth).[252]

Is the RTAC *Code of Practice* enforceable by law?

The RTAC *Code of Practice* intersects with some legislation so, if a particular breach or non-compliance is *also* prevented by Commonwealth or state legislation, the clinic will be considered to have broken the law. However, if a breach relates to *non*-legislative aspects of the RTAC *Code of Practice*, a clinic will only be required to take corrective action and will not be held accountable at law.

Are the NHMRC *Ethical Guidelines* enforceable by law?

The National Health and Medical Research Council (NHMRC) developed guidelines to be used by clinics, clinicians and researchers as part of their standard operating procedures but these guidelines are not legally enforceable. The Reproductive Technology Accreditation Committee (RTAC) uses the NHMRC *Ethical Guidelines* when accrediting and auditing clinics.

What are the repercussions of noncompliance with the RTAC *Code of Practice* and the NHMRC *Ethical Guidelines*?

Australian clinics are audited regularly. In all instances when a clinic is found to be *non*-compliant, the clinic must present a corrective action plan to one of the RTAC's independent certification bodies within a certain timeframe and a follow-up audit will be conducted shortly thereafter. Sometimes clinics undergo multiple audits—at their own expense—to ensure any matters of non-compliance are resolved. When nonconformity impacts patient safety, this must be corrected or addressed immediately. Then, based on the subsequent report by the certifying body, the RTAC can vary, suspend or withdraw RTAC certification.

Access to assisted reproductive technology treatment (ART)

In the past, certain people (for example, single women and members of the LGBTQIA+ community) were prevented from accessing ART treatment in some states of Australia. Commonwealth anti-discrimination laws would prevail if any such exclusionary state laws still existed, so any legal challenge would likely be successful.

In several states, other laws exist which outline standards a person must meet prior to accessing ART treatment (generally to ensure safety). Other than upholding the limitations described in these laws, clinics cannot discriminate on the basis of race, religion, sex, gender identity or intersex status, social status, disability, age, or reason for seeking treatment. Nor can people be denied treatment because they indicate they do not wish to participate in research (for example, donate their excess embryos).

However, there are some situations in which a fertility specialist may elect to defer or decline treatment. Possible scenarios include cases in which clinical evidence conflicts with the wishes of the individual (or couple), or when the procedure may have a detrimental effect on the patient or the child. A staff member or student practitioner at a clinic may also express a conscientious objection to participating in a particular treatment as long as, by doing so, they are not breaching anti-discrimination laws or compromising a patient's health.[253]

Location of ART treatment

The state in which the treatment took place will determine the legislation applying to each case. For example, if a person from Victoria travelled to NSW to undergo ART treatment, the ART legislation in NSW would apply. This can have direct implications for you and your child and is something to be considered at length. Such implications might include differing family limits, the age at which your child can access the identifying details of their biological parent and whether or not there is access to a donor register (see Chapter 15, 'Donor and Sibling Linking').

Reporting a birth

> *We donated our embryos and made agreements with the recipient about catching up annually, sending photos, etc. She was very keen and emailed us daily to check progress. After our embryos were transferred to her clinic, we didn't hear from her again. The clinic informed me she'd been unsuccessful, so I looked her up on social media and was shocked to find a baby photo that fit with the timing of the embryo transfers. I felt violated because we had put so much trust in this person, and to have that thrown in our*

faces was devastating. An investigation took place and new legislation was introduced as a result. I'm relieved that this little boy is now on the central register and will be able to contact his brothers (our children) one day if he chooses to.

Natalie Parker (Australian embryo donor)

Australian clinics are required to collect information about the outcomes of all ART treatments, regardless of whether a pregnancy or live birth occurred. This ensures that each clinic has accurate data about the number and sex of children born to a donor, any relevant medical details that might need to be passed on to the donor or other families, details of all parties involved in the birth, and the ability to pass on the information to the state's donor register. For the donor-conceived person born, it also means there is a record stating they are donor-conceived should their parent(s) neglect to tell them, as many parents were advised to do in the past.

Of course, this system relies on accurate reporting by patients (and accurate data collection by clinics). Sadly, even these days, not all parents are honest about donor conception or about the outcome of their treatment and there have been instances where women claimed they were not pregnant, when in fact they were. The Reproductive Technology Accreditation Committee recommends that clinics obtain a written agreement from intended parents stating they will notify the clinic of the cycle outcome. If a person fails to do this, a report will be submitted to the donor register (where applicable).[254] In some states, it is an offence for a person to provide false information to the ART provider about the treatment outcome[255] and, if a clinic doubts a person's report, the secretary who is officially in charge of the donor register can conduct an inquiry to investigate the intended parent's situation.

If you use an international donor, the requirement to report the live birth to the bank depends on the legislation and policy in that country. It's highly unlikely that anyone will enforce this but, in order to help maintain family limits and smaller sibling numbers for your child, it's vital you complete this step.

Birth registration and birth certificates

Registering a birth

In Australia, you are required to complete a birth registration form in order to obtain a birth certificate. Birth certificates are issued by the states and territories. The process only provides for up to two parental names and while legislation doesn't explicitly prohibit additional names, nor does it allow for it.

Birth registration forms vary between states and territories so, when entering your details (and those of your partner), you might be provided with various options such as, for example, 'Mother', 'Father', 'Parent 1', 'Parent 2', or 'Co-Parent'. In some states/territories, the birth registration form also requires you to indicate that the child is donor-conceived, but this does not mean the donor will be registered as a legal parent and gain parental rights and responsibilities. On the other hand, Commonwealth (and state) legislation indicates that if a person is named in one of the 'Parent' fields on a birth registration form, they are presumed to be the legal parent of the child[256] and Centrelink could pursue them for child support payments.

Solo parents by choice

If you are single and undergo conception at a clinic, you are required to leave the second 'Parent' field blank on the birth registration form. Depending on the state or territory, you may also need to provide the Registry of Births, Deaths and Marriages (BDM) with a letter from your clinic, or yourself, stating that you used a donor. A statutory declaration may also be required. Your donor's name will not appear on the birth certificate, they will have no legal responsibilities and they are not legally considered to be a parent of your donor-conceived child.

If you are single and use a known donor to undergo at-home insemination, all of the same principles will apply, except there will be no records of ART procedures undertaken with a donor at a clinic. Again, the BDM registries in some states/territories may require you to provide evidence, such as a statutory declaration.

Birth certificates

> *When I first found out I was donor-conceived, I spent months being angry that the government had allowed my most basic identity document to be a lie. I could not believe they would knowingly place the name of someone not biologically related to me on my birth certificate, and leave it there for my entire life without letting me know it was a complete fabrication and did not represent my genetic history at all.*
>
> **Australian donor-conceived adult (Vic.)**

Birth certificates play a fundamental role in maintaining accurate records of a population. Every human has the right to have their birth registered and to be able to access a birth certificate.[257] Depending on the country, a birth certificate can play an essential role in a person's life, impacting their right to vote, marry, obtain employment, open a bank account, access health services and education, receive an inheritance, and much more.[258]

Birth certificates are not necessarily proof of biology; they are proof of birth and evidence of legal parentage. Many donor-conceived (and adopted) people argue that failing to list the biological parent's name on a birth certificate is hardly a show of accuracy and, in fact, breaches their human rights by failing to identify their biological parents *and* an entire branch of their genealogical family tree.

After registering your child's birth, you will be supplied with a birth certificate. It might be possible for donor-conceived people to receive a birth certificate displaying the names of their legal parents and their biological parent(s)—that is, the donor(s). Check the laws which apply in your local jurisdiction.

Government benefits and child support payments

In order to be eligible for various government payments to assist with the costs of raising children, two parents need to be identified for the purposes of paying benefits.

But what if you've used a donor?

Two parents

If, at the time of an artificial conception procedure, you are a member of a couple (married or de facto; heterosexual or LGBTQIA+), as the legal parents you are entitled to any available financial support according to Centrelink's current criteria. If you separate at some point in the future, you may be able to claim child support payments from the other party.

Single parents

Submitting a birth certificate without a name in the second 'Parent' field can, on occasions, create havoc in the Centrelink office if the staff member has not been educated on the process required—and, yes, there *is* a process in place to deal with this scenario.

If you are single and use a sperm donor, in order to avoid Centrelink pursuing your donor for child support or maintenance payments, you must apply for a maintenance exemption—the intention behind this requirement is to prevent the government from paying wherever and whenever a person could pay.

Completing a maintenance exemption requires you to present a birth certificate showing you are the sole parent, as well as some additional documentation indicating you used a sperm donor. For instance, if you conceive via a clinic (in Centrelink terms, 'via ACP [artificial conception procedure] through a medical clinic or medical professional'),[259] your clinic will be able to provide you with the documentation necessary to verify that an artificial conception procedure took place. If you are single and you conceive via at-home insemination (in Centrelink terms, 'via self-administered ACP'), there are forms available online that can be completed by you and your donor as testament of your intentions. Alternatively, Centrelink might accept a preconception agreement or a statutory declaration. In that instance, you might need to meet with a counsellor at Centrelink to explain that you used a donor and that you and the donor are not co-parenting (you can even request this if you're having difficulty proceeding). Completing this process will also remove the need to explain your scenario to a consultant every time you make contact with Centrelink.

Subsequent to providing Centrelink with the required documentation, if you fulfil the current criteria, you will be entitled to the financial support available. Some people have reported being morally judged by Centrelink counsellors or have described the interview process as akin to an interrogation. If that is your experience, ensure you make a formal complaint.

> ***Note:*** Some people who have used known sperm donors simply lie to Centrelink and claim they do not know the identity of the second parent. This is usually done with the intention of protecting the known donor from being pursued for child support payments. However, if there is doubt, Centrelink may refer your case for an administrative assessment under child support legislation. In any event, it is unnecessary to lie to Centrelink and doing so could qualify as fraud or a dishonesty offence.

Legal parentage

Legal parentage is usually defined by whoever the intended parents are. When an individual uses donated gametes to carry out an artificial conception procedure, the gestational parent is considered a legal parent. When the gestational parent has a partner or spouse, unless they do not consent, they are also considered to be a legal parent. In Australia, the non-biological parent is not required to undergo second-parent adoption to be recognised as a legal parent.

However, the Australian High Court's decision in the case of *Masson v Parsons* [2019],[260] has blurred the lines when it comes to distinguishing between a donor and a parent—a person who donated gametes *may* be identified as the legal parent of a donor-conceived child. In other words, if the court sees a person who looks like a parent, behaves like a parent and is treated like a parent, the court will probably consider that person to be a parent. If the court decides continued contact with that person is in the best interests of the child, parental rights will likely be recognised and obligations and responsibilities will be imposed.

> **Note:** All legal cases are dependent upon multiple factors and the court judgment cited here will not necessarily apply to your situation.

Egg donors

When an egg donor is used, the gestational parent is considered to be the legal parent of the child, regardless of whether they are partnered or single (surrogacy exceptions apply). This is because the egg donor has already been through a legal process with the clinic.

Clinic-recruited donors and international donors

Clinic-recruited and international donors accessed via Australian clinics are required to sign documentation indicating they do not have an intention to claim parenting rights.

Conversely, intended parents sign documentation ruling out their intention to claim child support payments from the donors.

Known sperm donors

In the case of known sperm donors, recipients are not protected by documentation signing away the donor's intention to claim parenting rights. This applies even if you take your known sperm donor to a clinic or other medical centre to have them screened or undergo ART.

If you conceive via natural insemination (NI) with your known donor, this is irrefutably *not* an artificial conception procedure. The risk of undergoing NI is that, at any stage of your child's life, your donor may seek to be identified as the legal father of your child.

Co-parenting

For information about co-parenting see Chapter 6, 'Known Donors'.

Preconception agreement

> *How do you feel about co-parenting with your known donor? If the answer is a resounding 'No', then you might want to consider a different donor because if everything goes pear-shaped, this could be your life.*
>
> **Australian recipient parent**

The law applies equally to LGBTQIA+ and heterosexual families in Australia, however the rules tend to favour biology more than intention (especially in regard to biological fathers) and there are complex issues at play. In situations involving a known donor, it is highly recommended that you, your partner *and* your donor and their partner, seek legal advice and enter into a legal agreement outlining your intentions. It's important to be aware that donor conception is a niche area, so make sure your lawyer is well-versed in the nuances of donor conception—a generalist family lawyer *may* not be familiar with all of the issues. Legal documents may also outline the method of conception, and how many children you intend to have, as well as each and every aspect of your respective roles, responsibilities, finances, and so on.

The document does not necessarily need to be complex, but should outline the *intentions* of each person involved at the time they are signing the agreement—especially in multiple parent scenarios. The documents should also accurately define who is a parent and who is a donor, as well as provide clarity about contact. When aspects such as these are not made clear from the outset, or agreements are not observed, the risk of conflict increases. An example of a case involving a lesbian couple and a gay couple in which plans went awry after the child was born, despite there having been preconception discussions about co-parenting arrangements, is *Wilson & Roberts* [2010].[261]

> **Note:** All legal cases are dependent upon multiple factors and the court judgment cited here will not necessarily apply to your situation.

In Australia, the best interests of the child are the paramount consideration in all decisions related to parenting.[262] When determining the best interests of the child, the court will assess the particular facts and circumstances of each case individually, in accordance with relevant Commonwealth and state legislation. Legal parentage is only one contributing factor to the court's decision. A number of factors will be taken into consideration, including (but not limited to) the nature of the child's relationship with the donor or co-parent, the likely effect on the child caused by separation from that person, and any other fact or circumstance considered relevant.[263]

While a preconception agreement is not legally binding on a court, it is a contract outlining intentions and roles—making it an important piece of evidence that will be used to help the court reach a decision. The court may also consider any communications that take place between yourself and your donor so, from the outset, consider that each and every word you send via email, text, or other means, has the potential to become evidence in court.

Another important consideration when discussing and subsequently documenting your preconception agreement is to reach agreement on a process for managing disagreements between parties—particularly if you are in a co-parenting situation. This would include identifying from the outset the actions that will be taken to address any conflict, through the use of appropriate counselling or mediation with people who are skilled in this area. Ending up in the Family Court is an emotionally and financially draining exercise for you and your children and should be the very last resort. Even if you don't end up in court, the legal process is still draining.

Templates for preconception agreements can be found on the internet, although it's important to note that these documents may fail to cover your individual scenario adequately and frequently include inappropriate wording—including phraseology that conflicts with legislation and will, therefore, render it utterly useless in court.

When creating your preconception agreement, seeking assistance from a family lawyer who is well-versed in the nuances of donor conception remains the recommended option. Doing so could also save you vast amounts of money should your lawyer need to review and rewrite the erroneous agreement you downloaded from the internet.

Parenting orders

A parenting order is a binding directive from a court indicating the responsibilities and entitlements granted to relevant parties in a child's life. Parenting orders are not dependent upon legal parentage;

applications for parenting orders may be made by any person of significance to the child, such as a co-parent, a step-parent, a grandparent, your known donor, your donor's parents and any other significant people who are 'concerned with the care, welfare or development of the child'.[264] For instance, you and your donor (and their partner) might wish to co-parent.

The court will recognise and protect meaningful relationships with significant people so, where an adult who is not a legal parent has formed a relationship with the child, that adult could seek an order to obtain legal parenting rights. The order would stipulate: the modes of communication between the person and the child; and the amount of time spent; as well as other relevant directives.[265]

Parenting orders can be sought and granted with or without a court dispute.

Paying for gametes

It is a serious criminal offence in Australia for people to enter into a contract or arrangement to buy or sell gametes and embryos. This fact does not stop some donors from asking—and some intended parents from offering. Either way, it's useful to know that exchanging money for gametes could result in imprisonment.[266] Donors can, however, receive *reimbursement* for verifiable out-of-pocket expenses directly associated with their donation. This might include such expenses as the cost of travel and accommodation, medical expenses, legal fees, and loss of income.[267] If you are at all unsure, it is worth seeking legal advice.

The use and discarding of gametes and embryos

Human embryos are protected under Commonwealth law and clinics must have RTAC accreditation to create and manage embryos.[268]

Responsibility for gametes and embryos

For situations in which no legislation exists, the NHMRC *Ethical Guidelines* outline responsibilities and decision-making rights regarding the use, storage and discarding of donor gametes.[269] This might include scenarios such as a donor placing restrictions on the number of families who can use their gametes, the time at which a donor can withdraw consent, the reallocation of excess embryos to another intended parent or couple, and more. Check the laws which apply in your local jurisdiction.

Storage

All clinics must have policies in place for managing embryos. Ensure you check your clinic's policies prior to undergoing ART treatment. If you wish to extend the storage time of your donated gametes or your embryos, you *might* be able to apply to do so.[270]

Can I take my frozen sperm from the clinic to undergo ICI at home?

Taking frozen gametes home to undergo insemination is usually not permitted, because it creates a loss of control regarding data collection and subsequent control of family limits. There have, however, been cases reported in which a person has been able to take their unused gametes or embryos home for burial or to be made into keepsake jewellery, rather than them being discarded by the clinic.

Some clinics *might* allow ICI to be completed at home if all of the requisite processes, such as testing and counselling, have been completed at the clinic. Check with your clinic regarding the rules which apply in the local jurisdiction.

Importation and exportation of gametes

Within Australia

Gametes and embryos can usually be moved between states and territories of Australia, however approval may need to be obtained from both the sending and receiving clinic and there are criteria which may need to be met. Check with your clinic before making a decision about undergoing ART treatment interstate.

Outside of Australia

Gametes and embryos can be imported into Australian clinics if there is an existing service agreement with the relevant international egg or sperm bank.

When a person travels to a foreign country to undergo ART treatment, any embryos created can only be imported back into Australia if they comply with Australian regulation and ethical standards (for example, standards of altruistic donation, donor counselling and ID Release). People who travel to undergo ART treatment in foreign countries, where clinic conditions do not meet Australian standards, must return to that country to undergo further ART treatment with any remaining embryos.

Sex selection

> *Given the lack of understanding the layperson has of intersex variants, I think it is a dangerous idea to believe you can, in any way, ensure you have a child of a specific sex. As someone who is transgender, I also can't help but think of the obvious issues for a trans donor-conceived person who was 'purchased' as their opposite sex. At best, buyers beware but, at worst, this is a step towards eugenics.*
>
> **Terry Masson (Australian donor-conceived adult [SA])**

When it comes to conceiving a child of a certain sex naturally, a multitude of theories abound going back through the millennia and folklore provides us with many suggestions. These theories have also made their way into the realm of artificial insemination: turn up the hot tap in the bath for a girl and make sure you have an orgasm if you want a boy; inseminate before ovulation day if you want a girl, or *on* the day if you want a boy. While these theories are a little short on medical evidence, what if you *really, really* want a girl? Or a boy?

The possibility of choosing your child's sex raises all sorts of ethical and legal questions. Currently in Australia, sex selection is banned and, in some states, should a breach occur, legislation exists imposing a penalty of two years imprisonment.[271] The exception is when sex selection is used to reduce the risk of transmission of a serious genetic abnormality or disease known to affect a particular sex, and would severely limit quality of life for the child.[272] Check with your clinic about how to proceed if you believe you are eligible for sex selection for medical purposes.

Some countries do allow for sex selection for non-medical purposes. If you are considering this option, you might also wish to consider the impact that sex selection could have on your donor-conceived children if they discover later that you expressed a preference. Alternatively, in families where sex-selection by abortion has occurred [and clarifying that abortion as a basic right is not in question here], how will this impact a child who is born should they uncover this fact? Will the child feel pressured to conform to parental expectations regarding stereotypical gendered roles? What if your sex-selected child identifies as non-binary . . . or transgender? Will you be able to support them? And is there the possibility that a child's experience in this scenario might go *beyond* gender? For instance, some donor-conceived people express feelings of not meeting parental expectations because the donor's carefully selected characteristics do not match their own, or due to the lack of genetic connection and feeling 'wrong' in their family. Could the concept of having been selected in this manner amplify that experience?

In some countries where sex selection is allowed, some people destroy whole batches of embryos because they are the 'wrong' sex; others swap their male embryos with a family who has female embryos so they can each birth a child of the desired sex—yes, that's right, people are actually swapping their potential children.[273]

The topic of sex selection for non-medical purposes and its subsequent impacts is an ongoing discussion, incorporating a multitude of factors for the NHMRC and other ethical bodies in Australia to consider.[274]

Multiple pregnancies

You might recall the American woman, Natalie Suleman (otherwise known as 'Octomom') who gave birth to octuplets, even though she already had six children. It was discovered later that Suleman's fertility specialist had transferred *twelve* embryos into her uterus—eight of which survived. Her specialist later had his medical licence revoked.

Multiple births are considered to pose a higher risk for both the gestational parent and the children. Risks include: gestational diabetes, preeclampsia and postpartum haemorrhage for the gestational parent; and premature birth, low birthweight and developmental delays for the children. Additional care and ongoing support is required to eliminate or manage any complications.[275]

Australian fertility clinics are audited regularly to check for the incidence of multiple pregnancies. The RTAC *Code of Practice* recommends limits based on the age of the patient and the treatment cycle. For instance, when a person under the age of thirty-five is attempting their first treatment cycle, the recommendation is one embryo only. When a person is under forty years of age, the recommendation is no more than two embryos. When more than one embryo is transferred, clinics must ensure that patients are informed about the risks and hazards associated with multiple pregnancies.[276]

Donation from a relative

Let's say you're having trouble finding a suitable donor—can you ask your brother to be your sperm donor, or your sister to donate her eggs? What about your half-brother . . . your mother . . . your father . . . a grandparent?

Currently in Australia, there is legislation in some states preventing people from using gametes donated by a close relative. For example, in NSW, 'close' is defined as a parent, son or daughter, sibling, half-sibling, grandparent or grandchild.[277] In the absence of any legislation, the NHMRC *Ethical Guidelines* state that this practice requires special consideration because of issues such as undue influence by other family members on the child and the potential for the child to have confused family relationships.[278]

Of course, a woman or an individual who produces eggs and their close male or sperm-producing relative should not create an embryo together—and, while this scenario does not technically meet the definition of incest, it significantly increases the risk of passing on inherited disease. On the other hand, if you require a donated egg then you might use a close relative's egg and your partner or donor's sperm to create an embryo. If you are in a relationship and your partner creates an embryo with your close relative, that is a different story and many people do this successfully. It results in the child's biological parent being accessible and already part of the existing family and it also reduces the likelihood of multiple siblings.

Interestingly, cousins are a different story in Australia and, given a person is still allowed to marry their first cousin, or an uncle can marry their niece, there's no reason why a person cannot use their first cousin's gametes to conceive a child.

I'll leave that with you . . .

Family Limits

For more information on family limits see Chapter 9, 'Choosing Your Donor[s]'.

Part Eight: Donor-conceived People

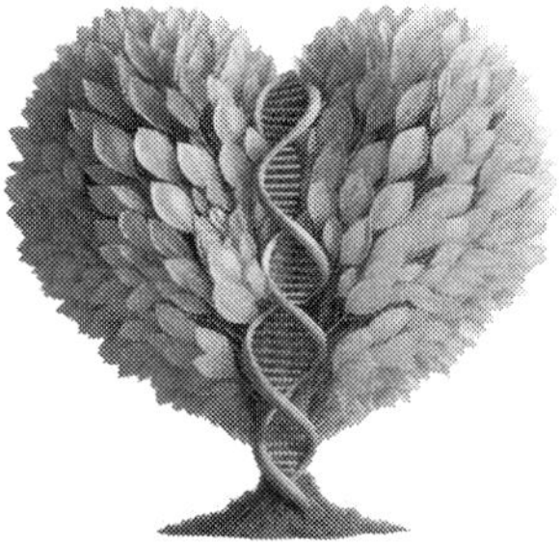

I greatly appreciate how they [my parents] *framed donor conception as 'my story' and how they supported me on my journey to find answers, even when they didn't fully understand why it was that I felt I needed to investigate further.*

Australian donor-conceived adult (Vic.)

If you've made it this far, you'll be familiar with many of the unique needs of donor-conceived people. It is my hope that this book has provided you with some knowledge, skills and tools with which to address those needs. This final chapter provides you with some personal insights shared by donor-conceived people; may their experiences help and guide you towards becoming the best parent you can be for your donor-conceived child.

17

Being Donor-conceived: Things my parents did well and things I wish they'd done differently

A 2021 study involving 272 donor-conceived adults reported an increased incidence of: problems related to identity formation; learning difficulties; panic attacks; alcohol and drug dependency; and higher stress levels.[279]

'Wait, what?' I hear you say. But this study is about *older* donor-conceived people—the ones who weren't told; the ones whose parents didn't have access to all of the information that we do, right? And there are now other studies telling us our kids are going to be okay![280] That the problems don't translate to our children—the new generation of donor-conceived people who know about their conception status from birth (hopefully) and are free to converse openly and easily with their parents about any issues that arise.

Right?

The reality is, it would be naive to assume all future crises have been averted because our children know the process by which they were conceived. Donor-conceived life is more complex and nuanced than just 'knowing'. Will our children experience pain? Will they be angry, sad, or indifferent? Will they feel fulfilled, impassioned or even overjoyed? Will they feel content about being donor-conceived, but angry about industry practices? Will there be some aspects they're fine with—and others not so much? Will they start off as indifferent teens and morph overnight into adults who shout from the rooftops about marginalisation and corrupt sperm banks?

The reality is that, when we set out on this path of conceiving a donor-conceived child, none of us can know.

What I do know for certain, is that we, as parents, have the power to influence our donor-conceived children's health outcomes. We can educate ourselves to make informed decisions, choose donors wisely and say no to unethical practices that might cause suffering to our children. I don't believe anyone intentionally sets out to harm their children, especially when we love them beyond measure but, sometimes, it happens. It happened to me.

And if, like me, you've already conceived a child who has dozens and dozens of siblings, or you selected an anonymous donor, or an unavailable donor who lives on the other side of the globe (or somewhere else), it's important to remember that you made the best choice available to you in the moment. So, if you feel the need, take the time to give yourself abundant amounts of love and self-compassion and move forward courageously with the knowledge that you will do everything you can to support your child to navigate their future path.

To help you (and me) along the journey, I asked a whole lot of donor-conceived people what their parents did well and what they might have done differently. Here's what they said:

> *I have always known I was donor conceived. We didn't speak about it often, yet when we did it was always open, honest and normal. My father was so perfect. He was loving, strong and taught me everything. He was my Dad. I was a confident, secure and happy child. Assets that have continued my whole life. When the time was right inside of myself I found my biological father. I was scared of hurting my parents. However my fear turned out to be irrational and unsolicited. My parents supported me every step of the way and encouraged me to be proud of every part of my being. Now I am more confident, more secure and happier than ever before.*
>
> **Kate Richards (Australian donor-conceived adult [Vic.])**

I wish my parents understood that my desire to know my biological origin wasn't a sign that their role as a parent had failed. They felt that I was criticizing them and wanted to exchange them with this new biological family.

Jasmin Sommer Alsholm
(Danish donor-conceived adult and Founder of Scandinavian Facebook matching site, 'Donorbarn—sæddonor—ægdonor'[281])

Mum never made me feel guilty for wanting to know about my biological father and where I came from. She always put my emotional needs first.

Australian donor-conceived adult (Qld)

I was a happy kid (and am a happy adult). I'll just say that I did not want to have any feelings about being donor-conceived as a kid. I knew my dad was scared it would impact our relationship. I knew my parents tried so hard and wanted to have a child so much. I did not want to disappoint them by being curious or caring about my conception. I still carry guilt about caring. I don't think I showed signs of this, but I do think meeting other donor-conceived people at a young age without parents present and having regular check ins and counseling would have helped me process better.

American donor-conceived adult

I have a great relationship with my mother, and when she expressed zero interest in learning about my biodad, it did feel like she didn't have curiosity or interest in what makes up half of me. She loves me and I know that, but it felt like she didn't have enough curiosity to know all of me which includes learning some information about her donor/my biodad, or showing some interest in who he is. She's since become open to that and it's really helped me talk more openly about it with her!

American donor-conceived adult

I wish I was told earlier so it wasn't a big thing. It made being donor-conceived feel wrong in some way, made me feel that I was wrong in some way.

Australian donor-conceived adult (Qld)

My parents did the absolute best job they could have bringing me up. They never told me (which wasn't ideal), but never gave me any cause to think I was any different to my naturally conceived brother. Having found out as an adult I am in awe of my father for keeping the secret that long and never ever letting me think I was any different.

Australian donor-conceived adult (Vic.)

I didn't like that Mum would make jokes when I was experiencing something like allergies or an illness by saying that I must have got it from the donor.

Australian donor-conceived adult (Qld)

My mum supported my need to know who my biological father was but left it up to me to find that information as an adult. It would have been amazing if she had tried to collect as much information as she could, even if that information was non-identifying. It would have also been good had she educated herself more about how to request information and the general systems within which donor conception occurs so that she could help me navigate that.

Australian donor-conceived adult (Qld)

I wish my parents had told me. I found out at the age of forty when my donor made contact with me through a government letter. If I had known sooner I would have had an opportunity to have a longer, more meaningful relationship with my biological parent and siblings. I am so grateful I know now, but I'm kicking myself I have missed forty years of relationships with my close family.

Australian donor-conceived adult (Vic.)

When I told my parents I knew, as an adult, I wish they were able to understand that it was a huge thing for me, but they were so caught up in it being a huge secret and stress for them and their whole infertility journey (which I don't minimise at all), they were unable to support me at all, at the time I needed them the most.

Australian donor-conceived adult (Vic.)

I wish my parents had been able to access groups/community for donor-conceived kids so that I grew up knowing other donor-conceived people but, perhaps, even more so to help normalise things for themselves by having contact with other recipient parents.

Australian donor-conceived adult (Vic.)

My mother is a truly excellent parent and the type of person I aspire to be. She genuinely and completely put me first. She never once tried to justify anything, never guilted me, never told me that something I said made her feel worse. She recognised that she made the choice to use a donor and part of that meant supporting me on my journey through what that meant. She spent hours talking to me, agreeing with me, listening to me. Any time I brought it up, she was ready to listen. She made it safe for me to express everything I was thinking and feeling. If you want to know how to best support your donor-conceived child, that's my advice. You have to give them a safe space to express ALL their feelings, not just the ones you want to hear.

Australian donor-conceived adult (NSW)

Don't ever stop talking about it [being donor-conceived]*, even when your kid is thirty-six years old, because it doesn't stop being their reality, ever. It's never 'over'.*

American donor-conceived adult

Conclusion

> *Would you tell me, please, which way I ought to go from here?* [said Alice]
>
> *That depends a good deal on where you want to get to, said the* [Cheshire] *Cat.*
>
> **Lewis Carroll (*Alice's Adventures in Wonderland*)**

When I sat down to begin writing this book, I did not envisage it would take me ten years. Had I known, I probably wouldn't have started. But something drove me to get up before the sun rose, to stare at a blank screen that needed words, to shed tears through a pandemic with a frightened child, just so I could get the word out about donor conception. Oh, what a complex topic it is—full of nuance, and differing perspectives and opinions! As a recipient parent in the donor conception triad, I continue to evolve daily with awareness and, while I may advocate for donor-conceived people, my privilege does not include supplanting the voices and the lived experience of those same people.

The good news is that you don't need to agree with everything that's written in this book—and only you can know which way you ought to go from here—but I do hope it has given you an understanding of some of the unique needs your donor-conceived child may face. Nevertheless, if something you've read in this book is causing you discomfort, I'd invite you to sit with those feelings and just see what comes up for you.

Parenting is one of the hardest jobs in the world (in my humble opinion) and everyone wants to see their children happy. Parenting a donor-conceived child brings with it additional responsibilities. So, if I have provided you with some concepts over which to ruminate, decisions to make, aspects to avoid, further resources to seek out and tools to get started, then my job is done. The rest is up to you.

If you have found this book useful, please share it with someone else. Give the book to another person who might be in need of a donor to build their family and ask them to read it. The world of donor conception desperately needs change—perhaps you will be responsible for initiating some of those changes. So get out there, start asking questions, talk to lots of people and assume nothing.

I wish you every success with your dream of building your family and may the next seven generations benefit from your knowledge and wisdom.

Oh, and don't forget to listen to donor-conceived people.

Why? Because you'll be raising one yourself.

Useful tools and resources

If you've enjoyed reading this book, please join my online community so you can access my posts containing additional resources, blog articles and the latest updates about donor conception.
Website: https://donorconceptionandbeyond.com.au
Instagram: @donorconceptionandbeyond
Facebook: https://www.facebook.com/donorconceptionandbeyond

Information about more tools and resources available to those undergoing donor conception is also available on my website (where the information can be kept up-to-date).

Social media (for example, Facebook and Instagram)

Social media groups and web pages about donor conception exist in abundance, especially on Facebook. I have intentionally not provided the names of specific groups here because groups on social media can be transitory, group names can change and some groups are more useful than others. And some groups, in my humble opinion, are probably best avoided.

If you do decide to search online, I can tell you that groups exist for virtually every aspect of donor conception you can think of—for example: infertility support; IVF support; LGBTQIA+ issues and support; donor-conceived teens; people conceived from donor embryos; donor-conceived adults; mixed groups of donor-conceived people, donors and recipient parents; sperm donor and egg donor support; known-donor families; recipient parent families; non-biological parents; non-gestational parent lactation; donor-conceived people who are also recipient parents; matching sites (both Australian and international); and more.

Terminology and language

When we discuss donor conception, we need to be careful that our language and the terminology we use is inclusive and respectful of all parties. Research undertaken by the LGBTIQ+ Health Australia, (formerly the National LGBTI Health Alliance) tells us that '. . . how we are described by others has an enormous impact on our health and wellbeing, as well as on how likely we are to seek health care when necessary.'[282]

The author has researched extensively and has had input from people representing all facets of the donor conception process. Her aim, at all times, has been to use language and terminology that is inclusive and respectful. Particular emphasis has been placed on the voices of donor-conceived people who are the only individuals who had no participation in decisions regarding their conception. Should any reader find offence in any of the content of this book, please be aware that this is unintentional and no offence has been intended.

Glossary of terms

To aid with understanding the meanings of some of the terms appearing in this book, explanations and definitions have been provided on the following pages.

artificial insemination (AI)

The process of introducing semen into the reproductive tract (cervical opening or uterus) with the intention of creating a pregnancy by means other than sexual intercourse. Some LGBTQIA+ people and their children dislike this term because of the implications of the word 'artificial' and prefer the use of 'alternative insemination' or 'assisted insemination'.[283] Nevertheless, given the term continues to be used worldwide, the decision was made to use it in this book to avoid confusion. No offence to impacted persons is intended.

assisted reproductive technology (ART)

A term describing a variety of medical procedures undertaken with the primary intention of achieving a pregnancy. These procedures include, but are not limited to, in vitro fertilisation (IVF), freezing of gametes and embryos, and the use of fertility medication.

biological parent

A term used in this book to identify people who are *genetically* related to their child. The author does acknowledge that carrying a child is a biological process encompassing more than just genetics and that the term biological mother/parent is also widely used by people who have used egg donors.

donor

A person who has donated or provided gametes (eggs or sperm) with the intention of relinquishing the rights and responsibilities of social parenthood. Depending on the restrictions imposed by the location in which the gamete donor donated, or their relationship with the recipient parent(s), the donor may or may not form a relationship with their genetic children.

donor-conceived person (DCP)
A description of a person based on the means of their conception or their genetic origin (using donated gametes). A donor-conceived person could have been conceived using a donated egg, donated sperm or a donated embryo. They may or may not have a relationship with their biological parent (donor).

donor-conceived siblings
People who share the same biological parent (donor), but do not necessarily grow up together.

donor conception triad
A term describing the three primary groups of people involved in donor conception: donor-conceived people, donors, and recipient parents.

donor register
A donor register is a place where information is held about the donor and the birth details of the donor-conceived child, as well as the person undergoing ART treatment.

double donation
When a child is conceived using two individually selected donors' gametes (egg and sperm), meaning the gestational parent (and raising parent) are not genetically related to the child.

embryo
An unborn entity created by a human egg and sperm, which has not yet reached eight weeks of development (after which it is usually termed a foetus).

embryo donor(s)
An individual or couple who have created embryos with the intention of donating one or more embryos to another individual or couple (or to scientific research). Typically, embryo donors create embryos for building their own family but have embryos left after they have completed the ART process. The excess embryos are then directed to other people who also wish to conceive a child. (Embryo donation results in the birth of full genetic siblings to the children of the donating couple.)

full siblings
People who share the same two biological parents. They may or may not grow up together. For example, people conceived via embryo donation

will be full siblings of the donors' children, as well as any other children conceived via the donated embryos.

gamete

A mature sexual reproductive cell. In other words, a sperm or an egg.

gamete provider

While the term, 'donor' implies giving without the act of payment, some countries pay their gamete 'donors'. As a result, 'gamete provider' is a term used by many parties to cover this discrepancy and describes an individual who is paid to provide their gametes, usually to unknown recipients via a commercial egg or sperm bank, or fertility clinic.

genetic parent

A person who contributed a gamete to conceive a child. A child's genetic parents can include the raising parent who contributed their genetic material, and the egg, sperm or embryo donors used by the recipient parent(s).

gestational parent

A parent who gestates (carries a foetus in the womb) and gives birth to a child. Genetic material may or may not be shared between the gestational parent and the child. The gestational parent is responsible for the nurturing and development of an embryo into a baby.

intended parent (IP)

A person seeking to receive donor gametes or embryos in order to conceive, gestate and/or raise a child. Genetic material may or may not be shared between the intended parent and the child.

jurisdiction

A country, state, or other defined area in which it is necessary to obey a particular system's laws or rules which are considered the authority.

legal parent

A person who has parental rights and responsibilities given by law, but is not necessarily a biological parent.

non-biological parent

A parent who is not genetically related to their child. For example, when a donor has been used. The non-biological parent may also be the gestational parent.

raising parent

A parent who is primarily responsible for the welfare and direction of their child's life and development. Genetic material may or may not be shared between the raising parent and the child.

recipient parent (RP)

A person who has used donor gametes to conceive and raise a child. A recipient parent may have also contributed their own gametes in the creation of their child.

social parent **(see: raising parent)**

solo-mum-by-choice (SMC) or solo-parent-by-choice (SPC)

Solo-mum-by-choice describes a mother who proactively seeks to be a parent without the presence of another raising parent, by using donor gametes.

The term, solo-parent-by-choice, is a gender neutral term preferred by solo parents who don't identify as a mother.

Endnotes

1 Rupnow, JM 2018, *Three makes baby: How to parent your donor-conceived child,* Rupnow and Associates Publishing, Dallas, TX.

2 Not her real name.

3 National Health and Medical Research Council, 2023, *Ethical guidelines on the use of assisted reproductive technology in clinical practice and research,* Canberra, p. 14.

4 Parker, AC 1916, 'The Iroquois Constitution', s. 20, paragraph 3, in *The Constitution of the Five Nations* (or *The Iroquois Book of the Great Law*), The University of the State of New York, Albany, NY, p. 39.

5 Victorian Assisted Reproductive Treatment Authority, 2021, 'Donor conception explained', *Understanding Donor Conception,* viewed 14 July 2023, <https://www.varta.org.au/understanding-donor-conception/donor-conception-explained>.

6 Darroch, F and Smith, I 2021, 'Establishing identity: How direct-to-consumer genetic testing challenges the assumption of donor anonymity', *Family Court Review,* vol. 59, no. 1, pp. 103–20.

7 Victorian State Government 2021a, 'Infertility in Women', *Better Health Channel,* viewed 12 July 2023, <https://www.betterhealth.vic.gov.au/health/ConditionsAndTreatments/infertility-in-women>.

8 Victorian Assisted Reproductive Treatment Authority 2023, *2023 Annual Report,* pdf, p. 16, Victorian Government, viewed 23 Nov 2023, <https://www.varta.org.au/resources/annual-reports>.

9 Rupnow, JM 2018, *Three makes baby: How to parent your donor-conceived child,* Rupnow and Associates Publishing, Dallas, TX, p. 53.

10 Ibid., p. 33.

11 Golombok, S, Jadva, V, Lycett, E, Murray, C, MacCallum, F, 2005, 'Families created by gamete donation: Follow-up at age 2', *Human Reproduction,* vol. 20, no. 1, pp. 286–93; and Golombok, S, Murray, C, Jadva, V, Lycett, E, MacCallum, F, Rust, J, 2006, 'Non-genetic and non-gestational parenthood: Consequences for parent–child relationships and the psychological well-being of mothers, fathers and children at age 3', *Human Reproduction,* vol. 21, no. 7, pp. 1918–24. These articles respectively describe the second and third phases of the research from a longitudinal study investigating whether children born through third-party assisted reproduction

experienced psychological problems or difficulties in their relationship with their mothers, as well as the impact on them of the disclosure of their biological origins.

12 Rupnow, JM 2018, op. cit., p. 60.

13 Victorian Assisted Reproductive Treatment Authority 2022, *Finding an egg donor*, pdf, p. 2, Victorian Government, viewed 14 July 2023, <https://www.varta.org.au/sites/default/files/2020-12/Finding%20an%20egg%20donor.pdf>.

14 Cusack, K (Health Complaints Commissioner, Victoria) 2020, *Inquiry into Assisted Reproductive Treatment practices in Victoria*, pdf, Health Complaints Commissioner, Melbourne, p. 33, viewed 14 July 2023, <https://hcc.vic.gov.au/sites/default/files/media-document/hcc_inquiry_into_assisted_reproductive_treatment_practices_in_victoria_report__3.pdf>.

15 National Health and Medical Research Council 2023, op. cit., section 5.6.1, p. 33.

16 Not her real name.

17 Bundesgerichtshof (Supreme Court of Germany), 28 January 2015, XII ZR 201/13, pdf, viewed 30 June 2023, <juris.bundesgerichtshof.de/cgi-bin/rechtsprechung/document.py?Gericht=bgh&Art=en&client=12&nr=70419&pos=0&anz=1&Blank=1.pdf>.

18 Victorian Assisted Reproductive Treatment Authority 2020, op. cit., p. 28.

19 Almeling, R 2011, *Sex Cells: The medical market for eggs and sperm*, University of California Press, Berkeley and Los Angeles, CA, p. 19.

20 National Health and Medical Research Council 2023, op. cit., pp. 25–6.

21 Cusack, K 2020, op. cit., pp. 10 and 43–54.

22 Fertility Society of Australia and New Zealand, Reproductive Technology Accreditation Committee 2021, *Code of practice for assisted reproductive technology units*, pdf, South Melbourne, section 2.8(a), p. 21, viewed 10 July 2023, <https://www.fertilitysociety.com.au/wp-content/uploads/20211124-RTAC-ANZ-COP.pdf>.

23 National Health and Medical Research Council 2023, op. cit., pp. 27–9.

24 Embryoland, 2020, *Embryo adoption in Greece: Successful and cost efficient*, viewed 14 July 2023, <https://www.embryoland.gr/en/pages/methods/Embryo_adoption.asp?fbclid=IwAR3o26kqXVPPxrsXgxmKAp6rprwKW9TwqVWXHsTKxDaP4_3cHomzf2TYdNg>.

25 Brennan, B 2019, *Single woman in Poland? Your embryos could be given to another couple*, ABC News, viewed 14 July 2023, <https://www.abc.net.au/news/2019-11-24/single-women-in-poland-embryos-could-be-given-to-others/11706842?fbclid=IwAR15wlhTLjlCyVA0nZ7vPtRUDa8tCOorjxjXEuR4qrWgmZltrEIzrEz3QVs>.

26 Fertility Society of Australia and New Zealand 2021, op. cit., p. 4.

27 National Health and Medical Research Council 2023, op. cit., 2023, pp. 24–5.

28 Ibid., pp. 33 and 34.

29 While the quote might or might not have originated with him, these words were used as the title of an article by Paul J. Killion ['Warning: The Internet may contain traces of nuts (or, when and how to cite to internet sources')], in *California Litigation: The journal of the litigation section*, State Bar of California, Sacramento, CA, vol. 26, no. 1, 2013, pp. 4–8.

30 Beresford, J 2018, 'Super sperm donor claims to have 'fathered' 78 kids from the back of his van', *Irish Post*, viewed 14 July 2023, <https://www.irishpost.com/life-style/super-sperm-donor-155214>.

31 Moses, C 2023, 'Man who has fathered hundreds is barred from donating sperm', *New York Times*, viewed 14 July 2023, <https://www.nytimes.com/2023/04/28/world/europe/dutch-sperm-donor-ban.html>.

32 Morton, N and Bell, S 2016, 'I fathered 800 children, claims sperm donor', *BBC News*, viewed 14 July 2023, <https://www.bbc.com/news/health-35262535>.

33 Lewak, D, Hauswirth, H and Beltempo, A 2019. 'Ari Nagel spawns 52 kids—and new "Sperminator" web series', *New York Post*, viewed 14 July 2023, <https://nypost.com/2019/12/05/ari-nagel-spawns-52-kids-and-new-sperminator-web-series>.

34 Victorian Assisted Reproductive Treatment Authority 2022, op. cit., pp. 5 and 8.

35 Ibid., pp. 5–6.

36 Lines, L 2019a (updated 2022), *Semen Analysis*, blog, Two Lines Fertility, viewed 14 July 2023, <https://www.twolinesfertility.com.au/post/semen-analysis>.

37 *Choice* 2016, 'IVF clinics and success rates', viewed 14 July 2023, <https://www.choice.com.au/health-and-body/reproductive-health/conception/articles/ivf-clinics-and-success-rates>.

38 Australian Competition and Consumer Commission, 14 November 2016, ‘IVF “success rate” claims under the microscope’, viewed 2 March 2024, <https://www.accc.gov.au/media-release/ivf-success-rate-claims-under-the-microscope>.

39 Virtus Health, 2017, *Annual Report 2017*, pdf, p. 36, viewed 14 July 2023, <https://www.annualreports.com/HostedData/AnnualReportArchive/V/ASX_VRT_2017.pdf>.

40 Cusack, K 2020, op. cit., pp. 9–12.

41 Royal, S 2019, ‘Woman who lost embryos in SA blackout tells of anguish as wind farm legal action launched’, *ABC News*, viewed 14 July 2023, <https://www.abc.net.au/news/2019-08-08/jo-postgate-tells-of-loss-of-embryos-in-sa-blackout/11393198>.

42 Boisvert, E and Rizmal, Z 2021, ‘IVF patients suing over inaccurate genetic tests find out some of their embryos were not discarded’, *ABC News*, viewed 14 July 2023, <https://www.abc.net.au/news/2021-07-06/some-ivf-patients-told-embryos-have-not-been-discarded/100270088>.

43 Fertility Society of Australia and New Zealand, 2022, ‘Vision & Objectives’, *About FSANZ*, viewed 14 July 2023, <https://www.fertilitysociety.com.au/about>.

44 Fertility Society of Australia and New Zealand 2021, op. cit., p. 5.

45 Fertility Society of Australia and New Zealand 2021, op. cit.

46 National Health and Medical Research Council 2023, op. cit., p. 11.

47 Ibid., pp. 14–15.

48 Fertility Society of Australia and New Zealand 2021, op. cit., p. 4.

49 Fertility Society of Australia and New Zealand 2022, ‘Board members’, *About FSANZ*, viewed 14 July 2023, <https://www.fertilitysociety.com.au/about/#board>.

50 Lines, L 2021 (updated 2022), *More on Success Rates*, audio blog, Two Lines Fertility, viewed 14 July 2023, <https://www.twolinesfertility.com.au/post/more-on-success-rates>.

51 National Health and Medical Research Council 2023, op. cit., p. 21–5.

52 University of New South Wales 2021, *Your IVF Success*, in association with the Australian Government, viewed 14 July 2023, <https://yourivfsuccess.com.au>.

53 University of New South Wales 2021, *Your IVF Success Estimator*, in association with the Australian Government, viewed 14 July 2023, <https://yourivfsuccess.com.au/estimate>.

54 National Health and Medical Research Council 2023, op. cit., p. 21.

55 Cusack, K 2020, op cit., p. 34–5.

56 Ibid.

57 Actual quotes from clinic websites.

58 Angelini, A, Francesco Brusco, G, Barnocchi, N, El-Danasouri, I, Pacchiarotti, A and Selman, HA 2006. Impact of physician performing embryo transfer on pregnancy rates in an assisted reproductive program, *Journal of Assisted Reproduction and Genetics*, vol. 23. no. 7–8, pp. 329–32.

59 Lines, L 2019b, *What is an embryologist?*, blog, Two Lines Fertility, viewed 14 July 2023, <https://www.twolinesfertility.com.au/post/what-is-an-embryologist>.

60 National Health and Medical Research Council 2023, op. cit., p. 21.

61 Ibid.

62 Dempsey, D, Power, J and Kelly, F 2022, A perfect storm of intervention? Lesbian and cisgender queer women conceiving through Australian fertility clinics, *Critical Public Health*, vol. 32, no. 2, pp. 206–16.

63 Ibid.

64 Lensen, S, Chen, S, Goodman, L, Rombauts, L, Farquhar, C and Hammarberg, K 2021, IVF add-ons in Australia and New Zealand: A systematic assessment of IVF clinic websites, *Australian and New Zealand Journal of Obstetrics and Gynaecology*, vol. 61, no. 3, pp. 430–8.

65 European Society of Human Reproduction and Embryology (ESHRE) Add-ons working group (comprised of K Lundin, JG Bentzen, G Bozdag, T Ebner, J Harper, N Le Clef, A Moffett, S Norcross, NP Polyzos, S Rautakallio-Hokkanen, I Sfontouris, K Sermon, N Vermeulen and A Pinborg) 2023, 'Good practice recommendations on add-ons in reproductive medicine', *Human Reproduction*, vol. 38. no. 11, pp. 2062–104.

66 Fertility Society of Australia and New Zealand 2019, *Use of adjuvants in ART*, pdf, Reproductive Technology Accreditation Committee Technical Bulletin 11, viewed 14 July 2023, <https://www.fertilitysociety.com.au/wp-content/uploads/Technical-Bulletin_Adjuvants-11-FINAL.pdf>.

67 National Health and Medical Research Council 2023, op. cit., p. 22.

68 Cusack, K 2020, op. cit., p. 9.

69 Ibid., pp. 9–11.

70 Newman, JE, Paul, RC and Chambers, GM 2019, *Assisted reproductive technology in Australia and New Zealand 2019*, pdf, National Perinatal Epidemiology and Statistics Unit, University of New South Wales, Sydney, p. 44, viewed 13 July 2023, <https://www.fertilitysociety.com.au/wp-content/uploads/Assisted-reproductive-technology-in-Australia-and-New-Zealand-2019.pdf>.

71 National Health and Medical Research Council 2023, op. cit., p. 19.

72 Cusack, K 2020, op. cit., p. 72.

73 Fertility Society of Australia and New Zealand 2021, op. cit., p. 19.

74 Cusack, K 2020, op. cit., pp. 51–2.

75 Words attributed to Jim Hawkins by 'Jonathan' 3 June 2017, *Accountability, healthcare: Misconceptions,* Reveal, podcast, transcript viewed 10 July 2023, <https://revealnews.org/podcast/misconceptions>.

76 Lindstrom, R 2020, 'Would anybody have paid him for his sperm?' Georgia Supreme Court Justices get heated deciding whether family can sue', *11Alive,* viewed 11 July 2023 <https://www.11alive.com/article/news/investigations/the-reveal/ga-supreme-court-hears-xytex-case/85-721a7948-d115-4f5c-a590-955d0f2042a4>.

77 Many of which are listed under *Is it Ethical?* on the website of the Society for the Promotion of Ethics in Reproductive Medicine (US), a subsidiary of the Donor Sibling Registry (US), viewed 11 July 2023, <https://sites.google.com/donorsiblingregistry.com/ethicsinrepromed/is-it-ethical>.

78 Brennan, B., 2019, op.cit.

79 Rupnow, JM 2018, op. cit., p. 89

80 Weiss, D 2020, 'Couple can sue sperm bank for misrepresentations; donor allegedly hid mental illness, inflated education', *ABA Journal,* viewed 11 July 2023 <https://www.abajournal.com/news/article/couple-can-sue-sperm-bank-for-misrepresentations-donor-allegedly-hid-mental-illness-inflated-education>.

81 Victorian State Government 2021b, 'Blood groups', *Better Health Channel,* viewed 12 July 2023, <https://www.betterhealth.vic.gov.au/health/conditionsandtreatments/blood-groups#rh-blood-factor-and-pregnancy>.

82 Buxton, Dr J 2015, *Can donor egg recipients 'pass on DNA' to their children?,* Progress Educational Trust, viewed 11 July 2023, <https://www.bionews.org.uk/page_95263>.

83 Ibid.

84 Blount, L and Jenkins, Prof. T 2021, 'How epigenetics plays a role in donor conception', lindsayeliseblount Instagram, viewed 11 July 2023, <https://www.instagram.com/p/CXEzkEDIevB>.
Tim Jenkins is an Assistant Professor of Cell Biology and Physiology at Brigham Young University, Utah, USA, and has completed multiple research studies in the field of epigenetics. In this Instagram video, donor-conceived parent Lindsay Blount chats with Professor Jenkins about epigenetics in an uncomplicated and accessible manner.

85 Inclusion and Professional Support Program (Australian Government Education Department) n.d., *Identity: A child's place in the world*, pdf, Community Connections Solutions Australia Inc; and Children's Services Central (NSW), viewed 13 July 2023, <https://www.acecqa.gov.au/sites/default/files/2021-01/IdentityAChildsPlaceInTheWorld.PDF>.

86 Gardner, T 2022, 'Why the donor's identity matters', *We Are Donor Conceived*, issue 3 *The After Life*, We Are Donor Conceived.

87 D'Arcy, C 2013, 'Costs of adoption: Genetic mirroring', *Musings of the lame, adoption & birth mothers: Building bridges to adoption truths*, viewed 11 July 2023, <http://www.adoptionbirthmothers.com/costs-of-adoption-genetic-mirroring>.

88 The Sperm Bank of California 2023, *Donor ethnicity*, Reproductive Technologies Inc., viewed 11 July 2023, <https://www.thespermbankofca.org/tsbcfile/choosing-ethnicity-my-donor>.

89 Stapert, E 2023, *Transracial adoption: Issues that may arise and tips to overcome them*, Manhattan Psychology Group, viewed 25 April 2024, <https://manhattanpsychologygroup.com/MPG-blog/transracial-adoption-issues-that-may-arise-and-tips-to-overcome-them>.

90 Heart Research Institute 2023, *Cardiovascular disease: Impacts and risks*, viewed 11 July 2023, <https://www.hri.org.au/health/learn/cardiovascular-disease/cardiovascular-disease-impacts-and-risks>.

91 Breast Cancer Network Australia 2023, *Breast cancer in the family*, viewed 11 July 2023, <https://www.bcna.org.au/understanding-breast-cancer/breast-cancer-in-the-family>.

92 Australian Government Department of Health and Aged Care 2022, *Haemoglobin disorders*, Australian Government, viewed 11 July 2023, progressively being updated.

93 The Fertility Society of Australia 2018a, *Age and reproductive outcomes*, pdf, Australian Government Department of Health and the Victorian Government Department of Health and Human Services, viewed 12 July

2023, <https://www.yourfertility.org.au/sites/default/files/2018-11/Age_and_reproductive_outcomes.pdf>

94 National Health and Medical Research Council 2023, op. cit., p. 31.

95 MedlinePlus [Internet], Bethesda (MD): National Library of Medicine (US) updated 2020, 'Is intelligence determined by genetics?', viewed 11 July 2023, <https://medlineplus.gov/genetics/understanding/traits/intelligence>.

96 Eren, F, Çete, AÖ, Avcil, S and Baykara, B 2018, 'Emotional and behavioral characteristics of gifted children and their families', *Archives of Neuropsychiatry*, vol. 55, no. 2, pp. 105–12.

97 National Health and Medical Research Council 2023, op. cit., p. 24.

98 Not her real name.

99 National Health and Medical Research Council 2023, op. cit., p. 31.

100 Ibid.

101 Ibid., p. 32.

102 McLaughlin, K 2017, 'One donor fathers 102 children in the Netherlands after giving sperm at 11 different clinics', *Daily Mail*, viewed 11 July 2023, <https://www.dailymail.co.uk/news/article-4819312/One-sperm-donor-fathers-102-children-Netherlands.html>.

103 *Our Father*, directed by Lucie Jourdan 2022, Blumhouse Productions, USA.

104 Cambridge Dictionary 2023, Cambridge University Press, viewed 13 July 2023, <https://dictionary.cambridge.org/dictionary/english/consanguineous>.

105 Kuznia, R, Gordon, A, Black, N and Lah, K 2024, ' "I slept with my half-sibling": Woman's horror story reflects loosely regulated nature of US fertility industry', *CNN Investigates*, viewed 19 Feb 2024, <https://edition.cnn.com/2024/02/14/us/fertility-fraud-accidental-incest-invs/index.html>

106 Fitzsimons, B 2020, *'Is this normal?' What happens when family members reunite and fall in love*, MamaMia, viewed 11 July 2023, <https://www.mamamia.com.au/genetic-sexual-attraction-personal-story>.

107 Harvey, J 2015, 'Blood money: Is it wrong to pay donors?', *The Guardian*, viewed 11 July 2023, <https://www.theguardian.com/lifeandstyle/2015/jan/25/wrong-to-pay-blood-donors-safety-compromised>.

108 Almeling, R 2011, op. cit., p. 12.

109 National Health and Medical Research Council 2023, op. cit., p. 26.

110 Ombelet, W and Van Robays, J 2015, 'Artificial insemination history: hurdles and milestones', *Facts, Views & Vision in ObGyn*, vol. 7, no. 2, pp. 137–43.

111 Monseur, BC, Franasiak, JM, Sun, L, Scott, RT Jnr and Kaser, DJ 2019, 'Double intrauterine insemination (IUI) of no benefit over single IUI among lesbian and single women seeking to conceive', *Journal of Assisted Reproduction and Genetics*, vol. 36, no. 10, pp. 2095–101.

112 Allahbadia, GN 2017, 'Intrauterine insemination: Fundamentals revisited', *The Journal of Obstetrics and Gynecology of India*, vol. 67, no. 6, pp. 385–92.

113 Lusignan, MF, Li, X, Herrero, B, Delbes, G and Chan, PTK 2018, 'Effects of different cryopreservation methods on DNA integrity and sperm chromatin quality in men', *Andrology*, vol. 6, no. 6, pp. 829–35.

114 Tober, Dr D 2018 (updated 2020), *The egg donation medical process: For egg donors,* blog, Fertility Smarts, viewed 11 July 2023, <https://www.fertilitysmarts.com/the-egg-donation-medical-process-for-egg-donors/2/1977>.

115 Li, Z, Wang, AY, Bowman, M, Hammarberg, K, Farquhar, C, Johnson, L, Safi, N and Sullivan, EA 2018, 'ICSI does not increase the cumulative live birth rate in non-male factor infertility', *Human Reproduction*, vol. 33, no. 7, pp. 1322–30.

116 Victorian Assisted Reproductive Treatment Authority 2018, 'Intra-cytoplasmic sperm injection (ICSI) and its possible effects on health', pdf, *Resources*, Victorian Government, viewed 13 July 2023, link located at: <https://www.varta.org.au/resources/information-sheets/intra-cytoplasmic-sperm-injection-icsi-and-its-possible-effects-health>.

117 Bhattacharya, S 2019, 'Breast cancer risk increased by IVF in women over 40', *Bionews*, Progress Educational Trust, viewed 11 July 2023, <https://www.bionews.org.uk/page_143534>.

118 Farhud, DD, Zokaei, S, Keykhaei, M, Hedayati, M and Zarif Yeganeh, M 2021, 'In-vitro fertilization impact on the risk of breast cancer: A review article', *Iranian Journal of Public Health*, vol. 50, no. 3, pp. 438–47.

119 Victorian Assisted Reproductive Treatment Authority 2018, op. cit.

120 Cavoretto, PI, Giorgione, V, Sotiriadis, A, Viganò, P, Papaleo, E, Galdini, A, Gaeta, G and Candiani, M 2020, 'IVF/ICSI treatment and the risk of iatrogenic preterm birth in singleton pregnancies: Systematic review and meta-analysis of cohort studies', *The Journal of Maternal-Fetal & Neonatal Medicine*, vol. 35, no. 10, pp. 1987–96.

121 Fertility Society of Australia and New Zealand 2021, op. cit., pp. 24–5.

122 Newman et al. 2019, op. cit., p. vii.

123 Victorian State Government 2023a, 'Twins—identical and fraternal', *Better Health Channel*, viewed 11 July 2023, <https://www.betterhealth.vic.gov.au/health/servicesandsupport/twins-and-multiple-births#risks-to-mother-and-baby-in-multiple-pregnancy-higher>.

124 Zhao, J, Yan, Y, Huang, X and Li, Y 2018, 'Do the children born after assisted reproductive technology have an increased risk of birth defects? A systematic review and meta-analysis', *The Journal of Maternal-Fetal & Neonatal Medicine*, vol. 33, no. 2, pp. 322–33.

125 Victorian Assisted Reproductive Treatment Authority 2021a, 'Preserving fertility', *Fertility treatment*, Victorian Government, viewed 13 July 2023, <https://www.varta.org.au/fertility-treatment/preserving-fertility>.

126 Pathology Tests Explained 2021, *Semen analysis*, Pathology Awareness Australia, viewed 11 July 2023, <https://www.labtestsonline.org.au/learning/test-index/semen>.

127 Mayo Clinic 2022, *Low sperm count*, viewed 11 July 2023, <https://www.mayoclinic.org/diseases-conditions/low-sperm-count/diagnosis-treatment/drc-20374591>.

128 Copp, T, Nickel, B, Lensen, S, Hammarberg, K, Lieberman, D, Doust, J, Mol, BW and McCaffery, K 2021, 'Anti-Mullerian hormone (AMH) test information on Australian and New Zealand fertility clinic websites: A content analysis', *BMJ Open*, vol. 11, no. 7.

129 Cusack, K 2020, op. cit., p. 11.

130 National Health and Medical Research Council 2023, op. cit., p. 22.

131 Services Australia 2022a, *Billing assisted reproductive technology services*, Australian Government, viewed 11 July 2023, <https://www.servicesaustralia.gov.au/education-guide-billing-assisted-reproductive-technology-services?context=20>.

132 Dempsey et al. 2022, op. cit.

133 Services Australia 2022b, *Medicare services for conceiving, pregnancy and birth*, Australian Government, viewed 11 July 2023, <https://www.servicesaustralia.gov.au/medicare-services-for-conceiving-pregnancy-and-birth?context=60092>.

134 Australian Government Department of Health and Aged Care 2023a, *MBS Online: Medicare Benefits Schedule*, Australian Government, viewed 11 July 2023, <https://www9.health.gov.au/mbs/search.cfm?q=fertility&sopt=S>.

135 Services Australia 2023, *Medicare Safety Nets*, Australian Government, viewed 11 July 2023, <https://www.servicesaustralia.gov.au/medicare-safety-nets>.

136 Services Australia 2022b, op. cit.

137 Mowat, A, Newton, C, Boothroyd, C, Demmers, K and Fleming, S 2014, 'The effects of vaginal lubricants on sperm function: an in vitro analysis', *Journal of Assisted Reproduction and Genetics*, vol. 31, no. 3, pp. 333–9.

138 National Health and Medical Research Council 2023, op. cit., p. 22.

139 The Fertility Society of Australia 2018b, *Parenting from before conception*, pdf, Australian Government Department of Health and the Victorian Government Department of Health and Human Services, viewed 12 July 2023, <https://www.yourfertility.org.au/sites/default/files/2018-08/Parenting_from_before_conception.pdf>.

140 Lines, L 2019c (updated 2022), *What's soup got to do with my eggs?*, blog, Two Lines Fertility, viewed 10 July 2023, <https://www.twolinesfertility.com.au/post/what-s-soup-got-to-do-with-my-eggs>.

141 Paffoni, A, Ferrari, S, Viganò, P, Pagliardini, L, Papaleo, E, Candiani, M, Tirelli, A, Fedele, L and Somigliana, E 2014, 'Vitamin D deficiency and infertility: Insights from in vitro fertilization cycles', *The Journal of Clinical Endocrinology & Metabolism*, vol. 99, no. 11, pp. E2372–6.

142 Gaskins, AJ, Chiu, YH, Williams, PL, Keller, MG, Toth, TL, Hauser, R and Chavarro, JE 2016, 'Maternal whole grain intake and outcomes of in vitro fertilization', *Fertility and Sterility*, vol. 105, no. 6, pp. 1503–10.e4.

143 Australian Government Department of Health and Aged Care 2021a, 'Folate and pregnancy', *Pregnancy, birth and baby*, viewed 11 July 2023, <https://www.pregnancybirthbaby.org.au/folate-and-pregnancy>.

144 Salas-Huetos, A, James, ER, Aston, KI, Jenkins, TG and Carrell, DT 2019, 'Diet and sperm quality: Nutrients, foods and dietary patterns', *Reproductive Biology*, vol. 19, no. 3, pp. 219–24.

145 Butterfly 2023, 'Risks and warning signs', *Eating Disorders*, viewed 11 July 2023, <https://butterfly.org.au/eating-disorders/risks-and-warning-signs>.

146 National Eating Disorders Collaboration 2024, *Eating disorder core skills: eLearning for fertility care professionals*, an initiative of the Australian Government Department of Health and Aged Care, viewed 3 March 2024, <https://nedc.com.au/professional-development/elearning/eating-disorder-core-skills-elearning-for-fertility-care-professionals>.

147 Purcell, SH and Moley, KH 2011, 'The impact of obesity on egg quality', *Journal of Assisted Reproduction and Genetics*, vol. 28, no. 6, pp. 517–24.

148 Håkonsen, LB, Thulstrup, AM, Aggerholm, AS, Olsen, J, Bonde, JP, Andersen, CY, Bungum, M, Ernst, EH, Hansen, ML, Ernst, EH and Ramlau-Hansen, CH 2011, 'Does weight loss improve semen quality and reproductive hormones? Results from a cohort of severely obese men', *Reproductive Health*, vol. 8, p. 24.

149 Victorian State Government 2021c, 'Weight, fertility and pregnancy health', *Better Health Channel*, viewed 12 July 2023, <https://www.betterhealth.vic.gov.au/health/conditionsandtreatments/weight-fertility-and-pregnancy-health#underweight-and-fertility>.

150 The Fertility Society of Australia 2018c, *Weight and reproductive outcomes*, pdf, Australian Government Department of Health and the Victorian Government Department of Health and Human Services, viewed 12 July 2023, <https://www.yourfertility.org.au/sites/default/files/2018-08/Weight_and_reproductive_outcomes.pdf>.

151 The Women's n.d., *Preparing for a healthy pregnancy*, The Royal Women's Hospital Melbourne, viewed 11 July 2023, <https://www.thewomens.org.au/health-information/pregnancy-and-birth/preparing-for-pregnancy/a-healthy-start>.

152 National Eating Disorders Collaboration 2024, op. cit.

153 The Fertility Society of Australia 2018d, *The role of exercise in improving fertility, quality of life and emotional wellbeing*, pdf, Australian Government Department of Health and the Victorian Government Department of Health and Human Services, viewed 12 July 2023, <https://www.yourfertility.org.au/sites/default/files/2018-08/The_role_of_exercise_in_improving_fertility.pdf>.

154 The Fertility Society of Australia 2018e, *Effects of caffeine, alcohol and smoking on reproductive outcomes*, pdf, Australian Government Department of Health and the Victorian Government Department of Health and Human Services, viewed 12 July 2023, <https://www.yourfertility.org.au/sites/default/files/2018-09/Effects_of_caffeine_alcohol_and_smoking_on_reproductive_outcomes.pdf>.

155 Pathology Tests Explained 2021, op. cit.

156 Ibid.

157 Ibid.

158 Australian Government Department of Health and Aged Care 2021b, *Smoking and tobacco and pregnancy*, Australian Government, viewed

11 July 2023, <https://www.health.gov.au/health-topics/smoking-and-tobacco/smoking-and-tobacco-throughout-life/smoking-and-tobacco-and-pregnancy>.

159 Australian Government Department of Health and Aged Care 2023b, *Quitting methods*, Australian Government, viewed July 11 2023, <https://www.health.gov.au/health-topics/smoking-and-tobacco/how-to-quit-smoking/quitting-methods>.

160 The Fertility Society of Australia 2018e, op. cit.

161 Victorian State Government 2022a, 'Pregnancy—medication, drugs and alcohol', *Better Health Channel*, viewed 11 July 2023, <https://www.betterhealth.vic.gov.au/health/healthyliving/pregnancy-medication-drugs-and-alcohol>.

162 The Fertility Society of Australia 2018f, *Sexually transmitted infections and reproductive outcomes*, pdf, Australian Government Department of Health and the Victorian Government Department of Health and Human Services, viewed 12 July 2023, <https://www.yourfertility.org.au/sites/default/files/2018-08/STIs_and_reproductive_outcomes.pdf>.

163 Jurewicz, J, Hanke, W, Sobala, W, Merecz, D and Radwan, M 2010, 'Wpływ stresu zawodowego na jakość nasienia' (translated from Polish: 'The impact of occupational stress on semen quality'), *Medycyna Pracy* (translated from Polish*: Occupational Medicine*), vol. 61, no. 6, pp. 607–13.

164 Prasad, S, Tiwari, M, Pandey, AN, Shrivastav, TG, Chaube, SK 2016, 'Impact of stress on oocyte quality and reproductive outcome', *Journal of Biomedical Science*, vol. 23, no. 36.

165 Victorian State Government 2022b, 'Absent periods—amenorrhoea', *Better Health Channel*, viewed 11 July 2023, <https://www.betterhealth.vic.gov.au/health/conditionsandtreatments/menstruation-amenorrhoea>.

166 The Fertility Society of Australia 2018g, *How to avoid chemicals that can reduce fertility*, pdf, Australian Government Department of Health and the Victorian Government Department of Health and Human Services, viewed 12 July 2023, <https://www.yourfertility.org.au/sites/default/files/2018-08/How_to_avoid_chemicals_that_can_reduce_fertility.pdf>.

167 Lateef, OM and Akintubosun, MO 2020, 'Sleep and reproductive health', *Journal of Circadian Rhythms*, vol. 18, no. 1, p. 1.

168 Victorian State Government 2023b, 'Pregnancy and teeth', *Better Health Channel*, <https://www.betterhealth.vic.gov.au/health/healthyliving/pregnancy-and-teeth#about-pregnancy-and-teeth>.

169 Almeling, R 2011, op. cit., p. 82.

170 Houghtaling, E 2021, 'I sold my eggs for an Ivy League education—but was it worth it?', The Guardian, viewed 11 July 2023, <https://www.theguardian.com/lifeandstyle/2021/nov/07/i-sold-my-eggs-for-an-ivy-league-education-but-was-it-worth-it>.

171 Martineau, P 2019, 'Inside the quietly lucrative business of donating human eggs', *Wired*, viewed 11 July 2023, <https://www.wired.com/story/inside-lucrative-business-donating-human-eggs>.

172 Foster, A 2021, 'Experts warn against murky world of private sperm donation in Australia', news.com.au, viewed 11 July 2023, <https://www.news.com.au/lifestyle/parenting/pregnancy/experts-warn-against-murky-world-of-private-sperm-donation-in-australia/news-story/c8e1b697cbb4566b4cdecabbd8e593db>.

173 National Health and Medical Research Council 2023, op. cit., p. 24.

174 Fertility Society of Australia and New Zealand 2021, op. cit., p. 20.

175 Fertility Society of Australia and New Zealand 2023, *Genetic testing*, viewed 12 July 2023, <https://www.fertilitysociety.com.au/preimplantation-genetic-testing-australia-new-zealand>.

176 National Health and Medical Research Council 2023, op. cit., pp. 51–4.

177 Tober, D, Garibaldi, C, Blair, A and Baltzell, K 2021, 'Alignment between expectations and experiences of egg donors: What does it mean to be informed?', *Reproductive Biomedicine & Society Online*, vol. 12, pp. 1–13.

178 Tober, D 2018 (updated 2020), 'Egg donation risk and recovery: What we know and what we don't', *Fertility Smarts*, viewed 11 July 2023, <https://www.fertilitysmarts.com/egg-donation-risk-and-recovery-what-we-know-and-what-we-dont/2/1980>.

179 Ibid.

180 Ibid.

181 Ibid.

182 Fertility Society of Australia and New Zealand 2021, op. cit., pp. 17–18.

183 Ibid., pp. 22–5.

184 Cusack, K 2020, op. cit., pp. 10 and 69.

185 The recipient and the sperm donor (hereafter known as 'donor') previously had a sexual relationship. After this relationship ceased, the recipient commenced a relationship with a woman with whom she underwent a 'ceremony of marriage' (not legally recognised at the time). The same sex couple wanted a child and asked the donor if he would provide gametes; they agreed that he would not have any parental role and would not

be responsible for the financial support of the child; the details were documented on a handwritten agreement. Conception took place via sexual intercourse in the presence of the mother's partner. The court cited the *Family Law Act 1975* (Cth), as well as similar cases, including several from the USA, to reach a decision which stated the donor was liable for child support payments.

186 Daniels, KR, Kramer, W and Perez-y-Perez, MV 2012, 'Semen donors who are open to contact with their offspring: Issues and implications for them and their families', *Reproductive BioMedicine Online*, vol. 25, no. 7, pp. 670–7.

187 Hertz, R, Nelson, MK and Kramer, W 2013, 'Donor conceived offspring conceive of the donor: The relevance of age, awareness, and family form', *Social Science & Medicine*, vol. 86, pp. 52–65.

188 Scheier, L n.d., *Considering egg donation? Here are six common red flags to watch out for*, blog, We Are Egg Donors, viewed 11 July 2023, <https://www.weareeggdonors.com/blog/red-flags>.

189 Ibid.

190 We Are Egg Donors n.d., *Interview: Inside Dr. Diane Tober's research on egg donors*, interview of Dr Diane Tober by Raquel Cool, viewed 11 July 2023, <https://www.weareeggdonors.com/blog/tober-interview>.

191 DNA Detectives is a Facebook genealogy group focused on using DNA to find biological family for adoptees, foundlings, donor-conceived individuals, those with unknown paternity and all other types of unknown parentage cases—recent and more distant.

192 Pascoe, Chief justice J 2016, quoted in: Victorian Assisted Reproductive Treatment Authority 2017, *Chief Judge John Pascoe on the child's right to know for the 2016 Louis Waller Lecture*, viewed 13 July 2023, <https://www.varta.org.au/resources/news-and-blogs/chief-judge-john-pascoe-childs-right-know-2016-louis-waller-lecture>.

193 Bloom, P (MB, ChB) 1957, 'Artificial insemination (donor)', *The Eugenics Review*, p. 207, viewed 12 July 2023, <https://www.ncbi.nlm.nih.gov/pmc/articles/PMC2973736/?page=5>.

194 Victorian Assisted Reproductive Treatment Authority 2023, 'Time to tell', pdf, *Resources*, Victorian State Government, viewed July 13 2023, <https://www.varta.org.au/resources/information-sheets/time-tell >.

195 United Nations General Assembly 1989 'United Nations Convention on the Rights of the Child' (UNCRC), Article 8, adopted 20 November 1989, entered into force 2 September 1990, United Nations Human Rights: Office

of the High Commissioner, viewed 13 July 2023, <https://www.ohchr.org/en/instruments-mechanisms/instruments/convention-rights-child>.

196 Jackson, E 2020, *2020 We are donor conceived survey report,* We Are Donor Conceived, viewed 11 July 2023, <https://www.wearedonorconceived.com/2020-survey-top/2020-we-are-donor-conceived-survey>.

197 Rupnow, JM 2018, op. cit., p. 54.

198 Kelly, F, Dempsey, D, Power, J, Bourne, K, Hammarberg, K and Johnson, L 2019, 'From stranger to family or something in between: Donor linking in an era of retrospective access to anonymous sperm donor records in Victoria, Australia', *International Journal of Law, Policy and the Family,* vol. 33, no. 3, pp. 277–97.

199 Rupnow, JM 2018, op. cit., p. 15.

200 Victorian Assisted Reproductive Treatment Authority 2023, op. cit.

201 National Health and Medical Research Council 2023, op. cit., p. 26.

202 Baden, AL, Shadel, D, Morgan, R, White, EE, Harrington, ES, Christian, N and Bates, TA 2019, 'Delaying adoption disclosure: A survey of late discovery adoptees', *Journal of Family Issues,* vol. 40, no. 9, pp. 1154–80.

203 Ilioi, E, Blake, L, Jadva, V, Roman, G and Golombok, S 2016, 'The role of age of disclosure of biological origins in the psychological wellbeing of adolescents conceived by reproductive donation: A longitudinal study from age 1 to age 14', *Journal of Child Psychology and Psychiatry,* vol. 58, no. 3, pp. 315–24. This research describes the research from the sixth phase of a longitudinal study investigating whether children born through third-party assisted reproduction experienced psychological problems or difficulties in their relationship with their mothers, as well as the impact on them of the disclosure of their biological origins.

204 Rupnow, JM 2018, op. cit., pp. 17–18.

205 Golombok, S, Jones, C, Hall, P, Foley, S, Imrie, S, Jadva, V 2023, 'A longitudinal study of families formed through third-party assisted reproduction: Mother-child relationships and child adjustment from infancy to adulthood', *Developmental Psychology,* vol. 59, no. 6, pp. 1059–73. This research describes the seventh phase of a longitudinal study investigating whether children born through third-party assisted reproduction experienced psychological problems or difficulties in their relationship with their mothers, as well as the impact on them of the disclosure of their biological origins.

206 Rupnow, JM 2018, op. cit., p. 44.

207 Ibid., p. 120.

208 Silverberg, C (author) and Smyth, F (illustrator) 2013, *What makes a baby?*, Seven Stories Press, New York NY.

209 Victorian Assisted Reproductive Treatment Authority 2021b, 'Telling children, family and others', *After donor conception*, viewed 13 July 2023, <https://www.varta.org.au/after-donor-conception/telling-children-family-and-others>.

210 Rupnow, JM 2018, op. cit., pp. 121–2.

211 Ibid., pp. 131–3.

212 Victorian Assisted Reproductive Treatment Authority 2021b, op. cit.

213 Ibid.

214 Mcleod, S 2018 (updated 2023), *Erik Erikson's Stages of Psychosocial Development*, Simply Psychology, viewed 11 July 2023, <https://www.simplypsychology.org/Erik-Erikson.html>.

215 Rupnow, JM 2018, op. cit., p. 135.

216 Persaud, S, Freeman, T, Jadva, V, Slutsky, J, Kramer, W, Steele, M, Steele, H and Golombok, S, 2016. 'Adolescents conceived through donor insemination in mother-headed families: A qualitative study of motivations and experiences of contacting and meeting same-donor offspring', *Children & Society*, vol. 31, no. 1, pp. 13–22.

217 Rose, M, Polcyn-Evans, J, Bergman, A, Azar-Tanguay, J and Bergeron, J 2022, *Donor conceived: A guide for people who have LGBTQ+ parents and were born via donor conception and/or surrogacy*, pdf, COLAGE, pp. 27–30, viewed 11 July 2023, <https://colage.org/wp-content/uploads/2023/02/Donor-Conceived-Guide.pdf>.

218 Rupnow, JM 2018, op. cit., p. 138.

219 Victorian Assisted Reproductive Treatment Authority 2021b, op. cit.

220 Jadva, V., Freeman, T., Kramer, W. and Golombok, S., 2009. The experiences of adolescents and adults conceived by sperm donation: comparisons by age of disclosure and family type, *Human Reproduction*, vol. 24, no. 8, pp.1909–19.

221 Dempsey, D, Nordqvist, P and Kelly, F 2021, 'Beyond secrecy and openness: Telling a relational story about children's best interests in donor-conceived families', *BioSocieties*, vol. 17, no. 3, pp. 14–16.

222 Victorian Assisted Reproductive Treatment Authority 2021b, op. cit.

223 Rupnow, JM 2018, op. cit., p. 69.

224 Ibid., p. 137.

225 Ibid., p. 133.

226 Rose et al. 2022, op. cit., pp. 33–4.

227 Ibid., p. 9–10.

228 Jackson, E 2020, op cit.

229 Rzeka 2021, 'Stop trying to find the "mechanism": The donor-conceived community is asking you to stop', blog, *Medium*, viewed 11 July 2023, <https://medium.com/@rzekameansriver/stop-trying-to-find-the-mechanism-196f5dc5cbf9>.

230 Rose et al. 2022, op. cit., p. 18.

231 Scheib, JE, McCormick, E, Benward, J and Ruby, A 2020, 'Finding people like me: Contact among young adults who share an open-identity sperm donor', *Human Reproduction Open*, vol. 2020, no. 4.

232 Fertility Society of Australia and New Zealand 2021, op. cit., p. 4.

233 National Health and Medical Research Council 2023, op. cit., pp. 59–61.

234 Ibid., p. 60.

235 Ibid., p. 33.

236 Victorian Assisted Reproductive Treatment Authority 2021c, 'Donor conception registry services', *Donor conception register services,* viewed 18 August 2023, <https://www.varta.org.au/donor-conception-register-services#:~:text=Donor%20linking%20is%20the%20exchange,is%20based%20on%20personal%20preferences>.

237 The Donor Sibling Registry, <https://donorsiblingregistry.com>.

238 Resnick, B 2019, 'The limits of ancestry DNA tests, explained', *Vox,* viewed 11 July 2023, <https://www.vox.com/science-and-health/2019/1/28/18194560/ancestry-dna-23-me-myheritage-science-explainer>.

239 National Health and Medical Research Council 2014, *Direct-to-consumer genetic testing: A statement from the National Health and Medical Research Council (NHRMC),* pdf, Australian Government National Health and Medical Research Council, viewed 13 July 2023, <https://www.nhmrc.gov.au/sites/default/files/documents/reports/statement-consumer-genetic-testing.pdf>.

240 *Teuscher v. CCB-NWC, LLC,* 2:19-cv-00204, (E.D. Wash.)

241 Donor Sibling Registry 2023, *Teuscher v CCB-NWB* [2019], 'Lawsuits', viewed 11 July 2023, <https://donorsiblingregistry.com/industry-issues#lawsuits>.

242 *Wilson & Roberts* (No. 2) [2010] FamCA 734. A lesbian couple and a gay couple, one person from each of the couples having known each other for

many years, and all of whom subsequently became friends, agreed to have a child together via artificial insemination. The men wanted to be fathers and actively involved in the child's life. Co-parenting responsibilities and time spent with the child were discussed and details documented. The men relocated from Queensland to Melbourne several weeks before the child's birth to be close to the child. Within months of the child's birth, the couples were disagreeing about time spent with the child, the women stating they saw themselves as the parents and saw the men as having performed no more than an incidental role. The couples underwent mediation which subsequently broke down. The men sought legal advice and the court found inconsistencies in the women's testimony. The women were given sole parental responsibility for the child and the men were granted access, the amount of time regularity increasing with the child's age.

243 These words were attributed to Maya Angelou by Oprah Winfrey (in 1995), and (in 1999) by Dr Phillip C. McGraw in his book *Life Strategies: Doing What Works, Doing What Matters* (Hyperion, New York, NY, p. 51).

244 Victorian Assisted Reproductive Treatment Authority 2023, op. cit.

245 National Health and Medical Research Council 2023, op. cit., p. 33.

246 Ibid., p. 24.

247 Fertility Society of Australia and New Zealand 2021, op. cit., p. 6.

248 Victorian Assisted Reproductive Treatment Authority 2019, *Regulator Plan*, pdf, Victorian Department of Health and Human Services, viewed 13 July 2023, <https://www.varta.org.au/sites/default/files/2020-12/2019-10-24%20Regulator%20Plan%20FNL.pdf>.

249 *Research Involving Human Embryos Act 2008* (Vic), Part 2 'Offences', S. 6.

250 Ibid.

251 *Prohibition of Human Cloning for Reproduction Act 2002* (Cth), s. 21.

252 Fertility Society of Australia and New Zealand 2021, op. cit., p. 5.

253 National Health and Medical Research Council 2023, op. cit., p. 18.

254 Fertility Society of Australia and New Zealand 2016, *Donation of gametes and embryos*, pdf, Reproductive Technology Accreditation Committee Technical Bulletin 8, viewed 12 July 2023, <https://www.fertilitysociety.com.au/wp-content/uploads/RTAC-Technical-Bulletin-Number-8.pdf>.

255 *Assisted Reproductive Technology Act 2007* (NSW) No. 69, S 62.

256 *Family Law Act 1975* (Cth), S 69R.

257 United Nations General Assembly 1989, op. cit.

258 United Nations General Assembly 2014. *Birth registration and the right of everyone to recognition everywhere as a person before the law: Report of the Office of the United Nations High Commissioner for Human Rights*, p. 6.

259 Australian Government 2023, *Guides to Social Policy Law: Family Assistance Guide*, '3.1.5.60 When maintenance action is not applicable', Department of Social Services, viewed 13 July 2023, <https://guides.dss.gov.au/family-assistance-guide/3/1/5/60?fbclid=IwAR3eQwpDSYVih4FqR6JZgKsep33exTeydXy-_W84T3YbVyzo0YssBwDdFeE#artificial>

260 *Masson v Parsons* [2019] HCA 21.
The mother and the donor (hereafter known as the 'father') had been close friends for many years and agreed to undergo artificial insemination to conceive a child. His name was recorded on the birth certificate. Although the child lived with the mother and her partner (note that they were not partners at the time of conception), the father continued to spend time with the child, have an ongoing role in the child's financial support, health, education and general welfare. He and the child were described as having 'an extremely close and secure attachment relationship'.
The mother and her partner sought to relocate to New Zealand with the child and the father instituted proceedings in the Family Court to prevent this from happening. At first instance, the Family Court found in favour of the father but, on appeal, the primary judge's decision was overturned. The father appealed to the High Court and, in a landmark decision, was found to be the legal parent within the meaning of the *Family Law Act 1975* (Cth). Factors the High Court took into consideration include that the father was registered on the child's birth certificate, that he provided gametes on the understanding he would be the child's parent, that he would care for the child financially and emotionally and that the child identified him as 'Daddy'.

261 *Wilson & Roberts* [2010], op.cit.

262 *Family Law Act 1975* (Cth), S 60CA.

263 Ibid., S 60CC.

264 Ibid., S 65C.

265 Ibid., S 64B.

266 *Prohibition of Human Cloning for Reproduction Act 2002* (Cth), op cit.

267 National Health and Medical Research Council 2023, op. cit., p. 32.

268 Fertility Society of Australia and New Zealand 2021, op. cit., p. 5.

269 National Health and Medical Research Council 2023, op. cit., pp. 36–41.

270 Ibid., p. 39.

271 *Assisted Reproductive Treatment Act 2008* (Vic), S 28.

272 National Health and Medical Research Council 2023, op. cit., pp. 48–50.

273 Ridley, J 2018, 'Couple hoping to swap girl embryo for boy may have found a trading partner', *New York Post*, viewed 11 July 2023, <https://nypost.com/2018/11/10/couple-hoping-to-swap-girl-embryo-for-boy-may-have-found-a-trading-partner>.

274 National Health and Medical Research Council 2023, op. cit., pp. 48–50.

275 Australian Institute of Health and Welfare 2023, 'Mothers who have multiple births and their babies', *Australia's mothers and babies*, Australian Government, viewed 13 July 2023, <https://www.aihw.gov.au/reports/mothers-babies/australias-mothers-babies/contents/focus-population-groups/mothers-who-have-multiple-births-and-their-babies>.

276 Fertility Society of Australia and New Zealand 2021, op. cit., pp. 24–5.

277 *Assisted Reproductive Technology Act 2007* (NSW) No. 69, S 28.

278 National Health and Medical Research Council 2023, op. cit., p. 31.

279 Adams, DH, Gerace, A, Davies, MJ and de Lacey, S 2022, 'Self-reported mental health status of donor sperm-conceived adults', *Journal of Developmental Origins of Health and Disease*, vol. 13, no. 2, pp. 220–30.

280 Golombok, S, Jones, C, Hall, P, Foley, S, Imrie, S and Jadva, V 2023, op cit. This research describes the seventh phase of a longitudinal study investigating whether children born through third-party assisted reproduction experienced psychological problems or difficulties in their relationship with their mothers, as well as the impact on them of the disclosure of their biological origins.

281 Site name translates from Danish as 'Donor child—sperm donor—egg donor'.

282 LGBTIQ+ Health Australia (previously The National LGBTI Health Alliance) 2013, *Inclusive Language Guide: Respecting people of intersex, trans and gender diverse experience*, pdf, viewed 13 July 2023, <https://d3n8a8pro7vhmx.cloudfront.net/lgbtihealth/pages/670/attachments/original/1587966204/Alliance_Health_Information_Sheet_Inclusive_Language_Guide_on_Intersex__Trans_and_Gender_Diversity_0.pdf?1587966204>

283 Rose et al.2022, op. cit. p. 5.

About the author

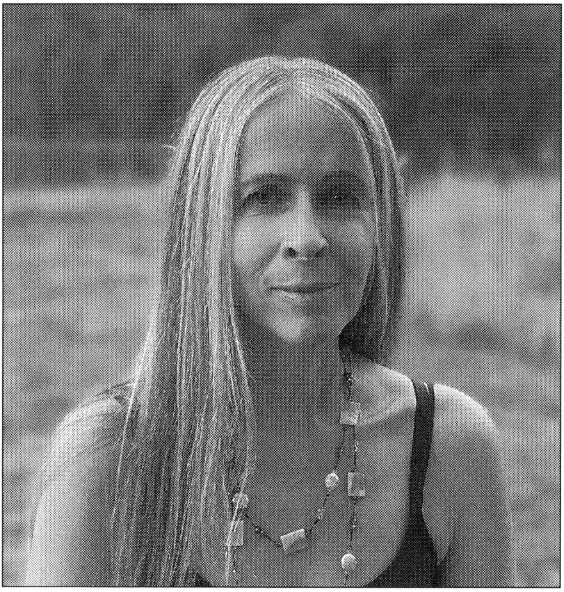

Gail Pascoe was born in New Zealand and relocated to Melbourne, Australia, at age two. After finishing school, armed with a Bachelor of Education from Deakin University she set off travelling the globe and developed a passion for seeing, tasting and trying new things; as well as enjoying the freedom to live in the moment and the joys of building lifelong friendships. After returning home and spending most of her professional career working for big corporations, she set out on her greatest, and most rewarding, adventure of all – becoming a solo parent.

Until her passing, days before the publication of this book, Gail resided in Melbourne with her donor-conceived daughter and a very spoiled Ragdoll cat.

Made in United States
Orlando, FL
04 November 2026

90201478R10219